Restorative Yoga Therapy

Restorative Yoga Therapy

THE YAPANA® WAY TO SELF-CARE AND WELL-BEING

LEEANN CAREY

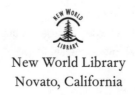

New World Library
Novato, California

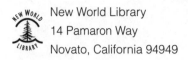

New World Library
14 Pamaron Way
Novato, California 94949

Photographs and text design by Wendy Saade

Library of Congress Cataloging-in-Publication Data
Carey, Leeann, date.
Restorative yoga therapy : the Yapana way to self-care and well-being / Leeann Carey.
        pages   cm
ISBN 978-1-60868-359-8 (paperback) — ISBN 978-1-60868-360-4 (ebook)
1. Hatha yoga. 2. Hatha yoga—Therapeutic use. 3. Mind and body. 4. Self-care, Health. I. Title.
RA781.7C358 2015
613.7'046—dc23   2015007680

First printing, June 2015
ISBN 978-1-60868-359-8
Printed in Canada on 100% postconsumer-waste recycled paper

New World Library is proud to be a Gold Certified Environmentally Responsible Publisher. Publisher certification awarded by Green Press Initiative. www.greenpressinitiative.org

10   9   8   7   6   5   4   3   2   1

I have been truly blessed with the opportunity to share yoga with gifted instructors and to learn from master teachers around the world. This book is dedicated to all the yoga enthusiasts who have entrusted me with their process and the yoga teachers who have given their time, knowledge, and invaluable life lessons.

Change is not something that we should fear. Rather, it is something that we should welcome. For without change, nothing in this world would ever grow or blossom, and no one in this world would ever move forward to become the person they're meant to be.

— B. K. S. IYENGAR

CONTENTS

ACKNOWLEDGMENTS

I extend special acknowledgment and gratitude to my family: Stephen, Robyn, Timothy, Alex, and Rob. For as long as I can remember, each one has supported me in my passion for yoga. I wish to acknowledge important people with whom I have developed business and personal relationships that have helped to make this book possible: Stephen Anderson, Jeff Homolya, Genesis Moss, Lisa Muehlenbein, Marc Newman, Wendy Saade, and Stacy Shimabukuro. I also acknowledge the book's models: the Carey kids, Yvette Hamara, Leilani Kashida, Jules Mitchell, Patrick Moore, Stacy Shimabukuro, and Marla Landa Williams. Huge gratitude and thanks to each of you.

I also wish to express special thanks to Wanda Marie, my spiritual sister, friend, and mentor and the greatest supporter of all I have ever tried or dreamed of doing.

My heartfelt appreciation goes to my editor, Ralph Cissne. I am grateful for the tireless effort he dedicated to seeing this project through and for providing an organized and concise platform for my message while remaining sensitive to my voice.

And my deep appreciation also goes to B.K.S. Iyengar, Donna Farhi, Judith Lasater, and Richard C. Miller, from whom I have received brilliant teachings on the art and science of yoga therapy. It is with utter gratitude and a humble heart that I stand on the shoulders of these teachers and many more who have taught me so much.

Finally, no teacher has influenced me more than Kofi Busia. His exceptional mind and honest perspective about the yoga community and the teaching of yoga earned him a uniquely honored reputation among students and yoga teachers. I am forever grateful for his presence in my life — on or off the mat.

INTRODUCTION

Yoga has been tested for thousands of years. It is more than an experiment or last resort. It is a proven path to wellness, healing, and longevity. It works.

There are eight limbs of yoga that serve as guidelines. This book addresses the third limb, asana (posture or pose). Each of us experiences challenges and triumphs on the mat. Our challenges may present themselves in flexibility, mobility, stability, clarity, or a host of other ways. I invite you to address the obstacles and opportunities you face on the mat with intelligence and a loving-kindness. This book provides the tools and understanding to meet these challenges with a unique practice that teaches we are more than our bodies and more than what we do. This simple yet comprehensive guide will prompt an inquiry about the level of support required to meet yourself where you are, a process that evolves over time. We simply need to be there.

Yapana is an ancient Sanskrit word meaning "the support and extension of life." Yapana Yoga Therapy is a physical practice that includes yoga props for strategic support to extend the life of poses, an extension that in turn supports and extends the nature of the experience. This style of yoga was developed on the basis of decades of experience in working with the physically challenged and with professional athletes, yoga teachers, and students — those with an inquiring mind who want to deepen their practice and balance their ego.

Let's take a closer look.

CHAPTER 1

YAPANA YOGA THERAPY

....

This practice meets people where they are. It is designed to encourage self-inquiry, reflection, and change, not perfection — the universe has already taken care of that part.

Yapana Yoga Therapy is a hatha yoga practice consisting of a series of simple movements to warm up the body, followed by DOING (dynamic) and BEING (relaxing) poses, held for an extended period of time with the support of yoga props, and ending with a STILL (final relaxation) pose to complete the practice.

This practice meets people where they are. It is designed to encourage self-inquiry, reflection, and change, not perfection — the universe has already taken care of that part. It is a gateway to discover how to apply its therapeutic outcome on and off the mat. The objective on the mat is to promote both balance and a positive and enduring effect while supported in both the heat-building and passive phases of the practice.

For purposes of this book, the BEING and STILL segments of the practice are deconstructed and explored. Oftentimes in a classical hatha yoga practice, yoga instructors and students value the stronger segment of the class more and, as a result, do not give ample time for the rest and relaxation phases of the practice. Because we live in a fast-paced world, restorative poses are a necessary part of our practice to help restore us physically, mentally, emotionally, and spiritually. We all require recovery time, some of us more than others. Incorporating this part of our living into our yoga practice will take care of the stressors that may lie ahead.

BEING POSES (SUPPORTED PASSIVE POSES)

BEING poses are the essential core of the Yapana practice. This is where the body/mind is supported into a state of relaxation and recovery. BEING poses give the body an opportunity to stretch passively and the mind the opportunity to experience what comes from doing nothing while supported in a yoga pose to elicit body/mind relaxation.

BEING poses are unique in that they help to stimulate the parasympathetic nervous system, often referred to as the "rest and digest system," which is responsible for the stimulation of bodily functions that occur while at rest. Although the body is in "rest mode," this does not always mean that the mind will settle into a quiet place. As with all other styles of yoga, however, practice and patience are the doorways into stillness and the settling of the mind.

The ample use of yoga props and their strategic placement are crucial to encouraging a peaceful experience in the BEING poses. One of the roles of the musculoskeletal system is to support the bodily organs. The better the musculoskeletal system is supported to meet you exactly where you are — stiff, flexible, or with a wandering mind — the more fully the body/mind can relax. When all urges to "do" are relieved, the body/mind can surrender and relax into doing less and feeling more.

BEING POSES ARE PERFORMED IN ALL CATEGORIES OF PRACTICE:

- Back bends
- Twists (seated, supine, and prone variations)
- Forward bends
- Inversions
- Miscellaneous (seated, side lying, supine, and prone)

BEING poses are held with support anywhere from 2 to 20 minutes. Refer to the practice timetable in chapter 10 (page 167).

I often hear from yoga students that practicing BEING poses has better prepared them for DOING, or classical, poses. And yoga teachers often tell me they learn more about the DOING poses while working with students and their own bodies in the BEING poses. This happens because whoever you are in any given DOING pose — however you avoid or overwork an area — presents itself quite loudly in the BEING poses. For instance, you can practice Utthita Trikonasana (Extended Triangle Pose) classically — standing upright in the middle of your mat. Any difficulties with front leg alignment, femur rotation, hamstring flexibility, or perhaps a neutral pelvis position will show up in the BEING version of the pose. But in the BEING version, you will have to address the challenges. The floor beneath you will prevent you from doing anything other than facing yourself, and so it goes with all BEING poses.

The support that is required in the BEING variation sheds light on what is or isn't happening when practicing the pose classically and can skillfully guide the outcome of any change necessary. BEING poses require little or no effort, meaning that they do not recruit the same level of muscle effort as DOING poses, other than getting into the pose and maintaining limb alignment. They are generally considered cooling poses.

STILL POSE (SAVASANA: CORPSE POSE FOR FINAL RELAXATION)

Savasana (Corpse Pose) is crucial to all styles of asana practices but especially to the completion of a Yapana practice. Because BEING poses have prepared the body for final relaxation, shortening or altogether ignoring this part of the practice would leave the student feeling incomplete. Savasana is a pose for integrating all that has come before. When we stop planning, organizing, and managing, we are able — if only momentarily — to experience the death of our doing. When this occurs, the full experience of a present moment's dying is only a breath away. Death teaches us that time and space are temporary and that clinging to life is an aversion to change. Savasana acts as fertile ground that creates an opening for the passing and going of all that keeps us bound.

In a Yapana practice, we allow a minimum of 15 minutes for final relaxation. Studies show that within that time, many people can drop into a state of deep relaxation, or what's considered the alpha state of mind, in which time and space become irrelevant to, or rather nonexistent in, your consciousness. As in all other yoga poses, levels of experience occur and change with time spent in Savasana.

Disturbances in this pose are not unlikely, even after a complete practice; they can surface from physical, mental, or emotional agitations. Everyone responds differently to a practice; however, both thoughtful and skillful sequencing of the Yapana BEING and STILL segments will encourage the greatest amount of rest with the least amount of effort.

How Would You Like Your Savasana?

There are many ways to take rest in Savasana, with or without support. Savasana does not have to be practiced the exact same way every time. Determining the kind of Savasana for the practice is based on what kinds of poses were practiced before Savasana. For instance, if the asana sequence addressed a stiff lower back, a logical choice may be to offer a Savasana that gives support to the lower back. If this is the case, consider practicing Savasana with either the legs elevated or weight on the top thighs to release the lower back into gravity. Or, if the sequence focused on opening the chest and shoulders, a logical choice may be to offer a Savasana that includes an eye pillow to support going inside.

Savasana as Preparation for a Pranayama (Breathing) Practice

Perhaps you offer a pranayama practice toward the end of the asana practice. If so, you may have taught poses that focus on opening the front, back, and sides of the waist and the chest and shoulders. Practicing a "mini"-Savasana (approximately 3 minutes) is recommended before a pranayama practice. This can help further mentally prepare for pranayama. Of course, after pranayama practice is completed, a full Savasana is recommended.

YOGA THERAPY — IT IS WHAT IT IS

Like so many others, I became interested in therapeutic yoga because at some point I understood that the value of an asana practice goes far beyond that of a physical workout. *Yoga therapy* is the new buzzword in the yoga community, but what does it mean? After all, isn't all yoga considered therapeutic? Yes, but in varying degrees.

All yoga is therapeutic, whether it is practiced passively or dynamically. What makes an intelligent yoga practice therapeutic is not one approach or the other, but whether the approach addresses the needs of the practitioners. Yoga therapy is not solely about practicing a relaxing yoga pose. It is about rightness: using the right pose at the right time, in the right way for the right purpose. It fulfills an intention, a purpose, and a direction. And it is a process and a road map for discovering what works for *you* while giving you the tools to integrate a vigilant understanding of how you do life on and off the mat.

After all, yoga (*yug* = to yolk, unite) is trying to teach us that its practice is not just about "me" (the ego) or what I'm trying to achieve (the pose, breathing practice, life skill, etc.). It is about joining the two in a way that is mindful, is meaningful, and extends well beyond the yoga mat. Simply stated, therapeutic yoga is about skillfully reconciling differences specific to your needs while drawing from the rooftop of your awareness to what is happening, while it is happening.

OVERVIEW — WHY USE YOGA PROPS?

B. K. S. Iyengar introduced props into the modern practice of yoga to allow all practitioners access to the benefits of the postures regardless of physical condition, age, or length of study. The central purpose for using yoga props is to address a need for support. Some people like to rename yoga props to sound more appealing, like yoga "toys" or "tools." I am not opposed to doing this, although personally I've never found the need. A "prop" is just that. It is supportive and helpful when facing obstacles on the mat because it helps to meet us where we are. That's the job it is intended to do. A prop is a prop. No amount of calling it something other than what it is will change the purpose. What will change is our understanding of props and their popularity, with intelligent, creative, and confident use.

Props help practitioners at all levels gain the sensitivity of a pose while receiving the benefits over time without overextending themselves. It allows students to practice asanas (postures) and pranayama (breath control) with greater effectiveness, ease, and stability. Still, some may be resistant to receiving support from yoga props because relying on props somehow diminishes their sense of success. If you have a negative attitude toward prop support, you may feel as though you are "cheating" in your practice and may generally oppose support in other areas of your life. Or perhaps requiring additional support shines a light on a shadow that you would prefer not to reveal. This I know for sure: if yoga instructors do not value using props, their students won't either. My experience over decades of teaching is that those instructors only lack the knowledge of how to intelligently and creatively use props. I wrote this book to help students and educate yoga instructors in how to use yoga props, to demystify them, and to inspire yoga enthusiasts everywhere to play and soften their edges on the mat with strategic and creative prop support.

We're ready to move forward.

WHO BENEFITS FROM PROPS?

Don't believe anyone who says using yoga props on the mat is cheating. One of my yoga teachers taught that asana practice is more about subtraction than addition (thank you, Richard C. Miller), and using yoga props can help every sincere student drop into that understanding.

It's perfectly fine to practice without the support of yoga props. It's just that in all the years I have shared yoga with different people at different levels of practice, I have yet to find one person who didn't benefit from using a yoga prop in one or more yoga poses. For everyone from the most flexible and strong practitioner to the least, a strategically placed yoga prop can elevate the physical and spiritual trajectory of the yoga practice.

In case you're not sure how this is so, I've highlighted how prop support can benefit yoga practitioners. Perhaps you'll recognize yourself in one of the groups below.

Yoga Newbies

If you are new to yoga, this book will help ease your way into the restorative journey. It will prepare you for practicing in a full-service yoga studio where use of yoga props is commonplace. Beginning students have much to learn. Prop support encourages students to investigate and organize themselves mindfully rather than following hard-and-fast rules of destination and time. This kind of learning fosters patience, acceptance, and self-reflection. These are the cornerstones of a mindful practice and one that has room to grow for a lifetime.

Yoga Enthusiasts

Let's say you're a yoga practitioner who practices a minimum of once or twice a week. Whether you are currently using yoga props or not, this book will help to refine your practice and develop your "inner" teacher. This book will help you to explore your physical and mental edges in a thoughtful way and can even inspire you to begin a home practice. Start by working with your favorite yoga pose, one that feels comfortable to you. Next, determine how long you can stay in the pose maintaining that level of comfort. Once discomfort surfaces, take note of the part of you that begins to tire. Feel your way into what's happening, and identify your greatest sensations.

Now try coming into the pose with prop support that allows you to maintain the pose a little longer, perhaps extending its comfort and shelf life for twice the time you had originally practiced the pose without support. Play around with the support until you are certain that it provides a level of experience that allows you to breathe smoothly and maintain safe alignment skills and a calm mind. Part of developing your "inner teacher" is to have a curiosity about what's happening "now" and to listen and follow your intuition. Your body/mind is brilliant. Your practice will speak to you in both quiet and loud voices. You only need to observe, listen, adjust, and wait. You'll be exercising the mind of your inner yoga teacher, an invaluable tool whether practicing by yourself or in a group class.

Yoga Teachers

Being of service through yoga is a rewarding experience. As an ambassador for yoga, you have signed up to practice, continue your studies, and spread the heart of yoga with others. This book will teach you how to see and teach your students, not just lead poses. Learning how to intelligently, skillfully, and creatively advise and adjust your students with prop support will enhance the overall quality of your teaching and their practice. Many students fail to discover the benefits of passive restorative yoga because their teacher may not be trained in that style. Learning how to use yoga props will open your students to experience a whole and balanced practice. A teacher who values the restorative side of yoga understands what lies beneath what's so obvious in a practice — that timing is valued over timeliness and process is valued over progress. These are just some of the rich lessons I have learned from my teachers.

You, too, can be this kind of teacher. The more you educate yourself on how to work individually with your students, the more yoga they will experience and the less ego they will fuel. Observing your students without yoga prop support paints a picture of where they can build and let go. Using yoga props to guide your students is a path to work within their limitations and safely maximize the benefits of a pose. This style of teaching clears the way for reconciling differences — yoga's ultimate path to freedom.

UNIQUE NEEDS

Weekend Warriors and Professional Athletes

More and more sport enthusiasts and professional athletes are integrating yoga into their fitness routine. Weekend warriors and professional athletes require considerable active recovery to balance the effects of intense workouts. Unfortunately, they don't always welcome a quieter practice. What is required after an intense workout is a slowing down from sweating and endorphin chasing, as well as a kind of mind that seeks stillness from doing nothing except feeling and breathing. Achieving this stillness is difficult for most of us but promising for all.

The BEING poses are particularly helpful to stretch, lengthen, and open areas that are typically overworked. A yoga practice that includes BEING poses promotes flexibility, an important element of injury prevention. Flexibility helps you to tap into your strength. Strength and flexibility go hand in hand. One without the other is like a table missing a leg — simply out of balance. In addition, a pranayama practice is an extremely helpful tool that fosters a stable, calm, and present state of mind and can translate into improving your athletic performance and sharpening your ability to focus.

Yoga Practitioners with Injuries

An intelligent yoga practice can address a host of physical, emotional, and spiritual concerns. Ancient yoga philosophy states that each of us is made of five koshas (sheaths): physicality, energy (breath or life force), mind (intellect), perception (intuition, wisdom), and spirit (innate joy, peace, and harmony). My yoga practice has proved to me that these layers are connected much as the anklebone is connected to the hip bone. Although the two bones may not be directly connected, if one is affected the other may likely be as well. Since yoga therapists are not doctors, treating any chronic condition with certainty can be risky; however, yogic principles and therapies that have proved successful can be applied wisely using a basic tried-and-true balanced approach, including most or all of the following:

• Relaxation
• Traction (if there is compression)
• Mobilization
• Stabilization and strengthening

For decades I have used this simple approach with yoga students to help them manage and recover from injuries. It doesn't mean that students with severe issues can avoid necessary surgery. However, I have prescribed many combinations of these yoga therapies using this approach, which can include both DOING and BEING poses or one or the other, all practiced with yoga prop support, to prepare students for presurgery and to speed up the recovery time postsurgery. Again, I can't stress enough how important it is to link all "layers" for holistic healing and productive injury management.

Massage Therapists

If you are a massage therapist, you may already be stretching your clients. In my opinion, integrating massage with a few targeted BEING poses that address your clients' habitual holding patterns is a perfect recipe for deep letting-go. Being supported in a passive yoga pose by both gravity and strategically placed yoga props is a unique experience. It always encourages a deep level of relaxation that may otherwise be difficult to access through assisted stretching. Here, there is nothing to do and nowhere to go. Your clients can be suspended in the experience of a yoga prop–supported stretch while breathing, feeling, sensing, and letting go. Sounds good, right?

CHAPTER 2

MEET YOUR YOGA PROPS

....

That which I seek finds me, embraces me, and knows me.
It lives inside me.

Each of the yoga props listed in this chapter (except for the eye pillow) can be used in practice in all classifications of yoga poses — standing, seated, back bending, twisting, inverting, and forward bending — whether they are DOING or BEING poses. I have my personal prop preferences in style, size, material, and manufacturer. If you are a budget-minded yogi, however, the expense of yoga props shouldn't deter you from creating an ample prop inventory. When I first started teaching, I used books for blocks, towels for blankets, couch cushions for bolsters, dining room chairs for support, fabric remnants sewed together for belts (trust me, I am *not* a seamstress!), and a kitchen sink and door jams for leverage (yes, even a kitchen sink!). All is possible. All the time. Always. Think outside the box.

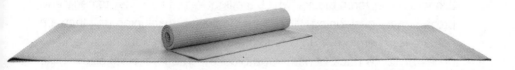

Yoga Mat

Yoga mat manufacturers produce mats in various thicknesses. For ample support, whether the mat requires folding or rolling, it should measure no more than $3/16$ inch deep, and I prefer a nonskid mat for sufficient stickiness. This guarantees the holding in place of other yoga props that may be used in combination with the mat. Check out local yoga studios that may be replacing old mats. You might be able to purchase used mats for a buck or two. Just clean the you-know-what out of them, and use them for props. Consider reaching out to your yoga buddies to see if they have an extra mat they no longer use because they don't like it. The plethora of mats I've collected over the years includes expensive mats people have purchased but didn't like for one reason or another. If I can't use the entire mat as a prop, I cut it up into various-sized square sheets and use them as pads for bony body parts and lifts for feet. Get creative!

HOW TO USE: Yoga mats can cushion bony body parts; hold blocks, blankets, bolsters, and chairs in place; or be rolled up into tubes as a substitute for blankets or bolsters. The best yoga mats for use as props are quite sticky, can easily roll, and are not too thick. The wonderful thick mats that are now on the market are great for lying and practicing, but they are often far too thick to use as props.

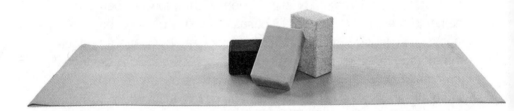

Blocks

I prefer cork blocks because of their unique combination of stability, weight, and ability to slide against the floor when necessary. Some practitioners prefer foam blocks, which are lightweight and easy to carry and provide more cushioning. I like foam blocks for cushioning, but they are not stable. Therefore, I don't recommend them for supporting standing poses or some back bends. Yoga blocks come in several sizes. I like the standard size, which is 4 x 6 x 9 inches. Having a few different sizes, however, is convenient. Sometimes a student needs a 4 x 6 x 9-inch block and another block half that thick. Blocks can be placed in three different ways, resulting in three possible heights: they can be laid flat (lowest height), placed on edge (middle height), or stood on end (tallest height). If you don't have a block, consider using a book, preferably one you've already read so you don't get distracted.

HOW TO USE: Blocks can be used to bring the floor to you to assist with flexibility or to wake up dull areas of your body. They also help to "reduce the reach," access core stability, and provide unique leverage in far-reaching forward bends. Blocks are very versatile, and you will love them.

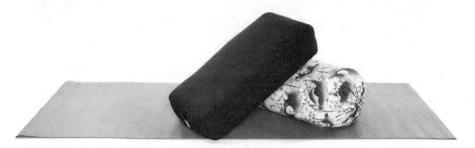

Bolster

Bolsters come in all sizes and shapes. Finding the right-sized bolster for you is important. If you are petite like me, a bolster that is half your body size doesn't always work. Too much support isn't helpful, and not enough doesn't serve the purpose. I recommend you begin with a standard-sized bolster. You can always add folded blankets on top to create more height when needed. The most commonly used bolster is a standard "flat" bolster, measuring 8 x 27 x 32.5 inches and weighing 5 pounds. An oval bolster, measuring 9 x 26 x 34.5 inches, weighs 7 pounds. Choosing the right bolster for each pose and each person depends on the level of support individually needed and how the bolster best supports the trajectory of the pose.

HOW TO USE: In short, bolsters do exactly what their name suggests — they bolster a part of the body in order to open, release, or support that part. They are truly a godsend.

Wall

For vertical support, use a clean, sturdy, and flat wall without glass or a mirror. Besides a chair, a wall is my favorite yoga prop. You can push against, relax into, leverage from, and confront your fears with its support. Everyone has a wall in his or her house, yoga studio, or gym. Do not use a mirrored wall unless that's all you have, in which case proceed with caution. I don't recommend flipping up into a handstand on a mirrored wall unless you are certain of its stability and security. When using a chair against a mirrored wall, simply pad the back reinforcement bar of the chair with a blanket to prevent scratching or breaking the mirror. In a pinch, you can use a securely closed door with a flat surface. Also, a corner where two walls meet provides excellent alignment feedback for either side of the body. Try it and notice what you feel.

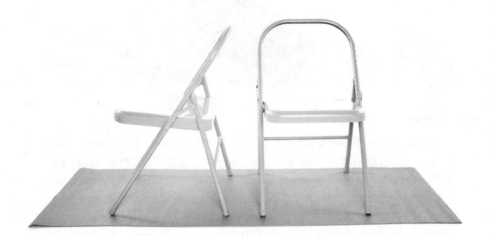

Chair or Stool

You can use a sturdy folding chair with a reinforcement bar in the back but with the backrest of the chair pushed out. If you hammer out the chair's backrest, be sure to file any rough edges. Another option is to wrap the back of the chair frame with athletic tape. I learned that nifty trick from one of the Yapana Yoga mentors, and it works well because it also offers a nice grip for your hands. I learned my lesson working with athletes up to 6 feet 9 inches tall. The standard folding chair is too short (thanks, Luke!). In this case, it might be best in some yoga poses to use a stool or to prop your chair on blocks to make it taller. When working in a gym environment, I like stacking aerobic steps, because they provide a stable seat that sometimes a stool does not. And there is a new folding chair on the market that extends the normal height up to six inches. There isn't an excuse not to use one.

HOW TO USE: The chair is another favorite yoga prop of mine, as it can provide a little more "restful" support. When necessary, you can drop all of your body weight onto the seat surface. I've included some very creative approaches to poses with the support of a chair. Note: sometimes you need to position the chair next to a wall so that it doesn't move.

Blankets

Be particular about your blankets. The ones made entirely out of polyester are difficult to fold, and those that are strictly wool generate a funky smell after continued use and care. What to do? Purchase blankets that are a mix of the two materials. If you want to avoid the expense, use ones that you can afford and are readily available. Even folded up blankets from your house or bath or beach towels will work. Use what works for you and provides the level of support needed.

HOW TO USE: Blankets can be used to bring the floor to you, to cushion hard areas, and to weigh down an area of the body to help it release. Rolled or folded, they provide excellent support for chest openers, twists, and forward bends. Some BEING poses require short- or long-rolled blankets or double- or accordion-folded blankets. No matter which style of fold you use, always roll and fold the blankets so they have clean edges as they are supporting your body weight. Blankets fall apart when they are not carefully folded, and this will affect the level of support they provide.

Many folds and rolls begin with a single-folded blanket, called Foundation. From this shape you can make just about any of the other required shapes.

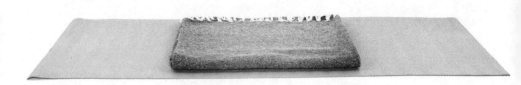

HOW TO FOLD A SINGLE-FOLDED BLANKET — FOUNDATION

1. Starting with the short ends of a blanket, fold it in half.
2. From the short ends, fold it in half again two more times.
3. Smooth out any wrinkles, and align the edges.

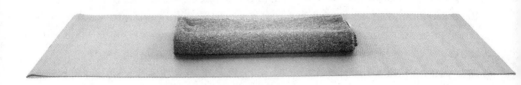

HOW TO FOLD A DOUBLE-FOLDED BLANKET

1. Start with a Foundation blanket shape.
2. Fold it in half from the long, clean edges.
3. Smooth out any wrinkles, and align the edges.

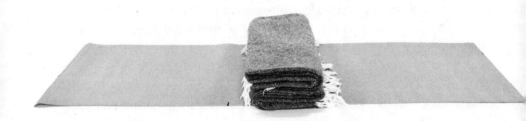

HOW TO FOLD TWO DOUBLE-FOLDED STACKED BLANKETS (AS A BOLSTER)

1. Stack two double-folded blankets so that their clean edges align with each other.
2. Smooth out any wrinkles, and align all edges.

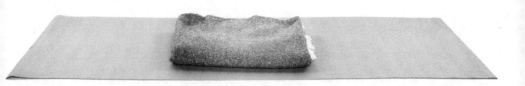

HOW TO FOLD A MEDITATION PAD BLANKET

1. Start with a Foundation blanket shape.
2. From the short clean edge, fold in half.
3. Smooth out any wrinkles, and align the edges.

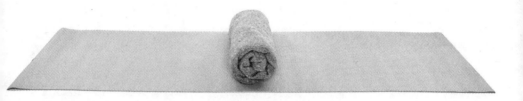

HOW TO ROLL A SHORT-ROLLED BLANKET

1. Start with a Foundation blanket shape.
2. From the short clean edge, tightly roll into a solid cylinder.
3. Smooth out any wrinkles, and align the edges.

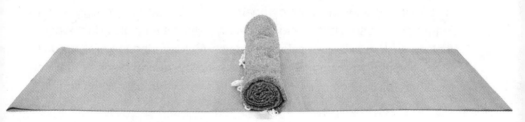

HOW TO ROLL A LONG-ROLLED BLANKET

1. Start with a Foundation blanket shape.
2. From the long clean edge, tightly roll into a solid cylinder.
3. Smooth out any wrinkles, and align the edges.

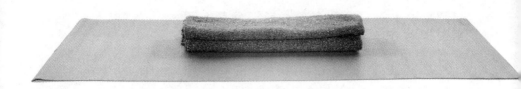

HOW TO FOLD AN ACCORDION-FOLDED BLANKET

1. Start with a Foundation blanket shape.
2. From the long clean edge, fold in quarters accordion style.
3. Smooth out any wrinkles, and align the edges.

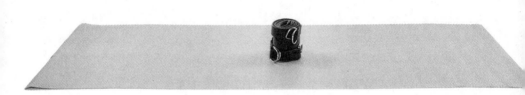

Belt

Belts also come in many sizes. I prefer using 10-foot belts because they provide the most options. It's better to have a belt that's too long than one that's too short. If too short, you have to tie belts together to make a long one, which is confusing. The difference in the prices of a 6-foot belt and a 10-foot belt is insignificant compared to the benefits of working with a longer one. I also recommend the D-ring belts, as they provide the best locking system and are easiest to adjust. Although the long D-ring belt is my favorite, you can make a similar prop by sewing pieces of fabric together. But I encourage you to invest in a real yoga belt. When you do, you won't be sorry.

HOW TO USE: Belts stabilize joints, encourage flexibility, support inflexible parts of the body, and create traction and space — two magic words in yoga therapy, as many suffer compression somewhere. Using a yoga belt can provide instant relief for some people. Need I say more?

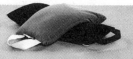

Sandbag

The sandbag is another genius idea from B. K. S. Iyengar. It's a yoga prop that provides weight and encourages overworked areas to release. Yapana therapy students are hooked on sandbags. Classical weight plates were once used, the old-school kind that are still used in gyms. Imagine being in Savasana (Corpse Pose) with a few large round weights stacked on top of the pelvis and legs. Don't laugh until you try it. I'll try just about anything that I think might provide the kind of support I need at any given time. However, sandbags work even better than weight plates, and you can make your own. Whether you use sand (don't steal it from the beach; buy it from the store), pea gravel, rice, or some other substance for the bag, be sure you do not entirely fill the bag, because it needs to be manipulable so that you can rest only part of it on a limb if needed.

SANDBAG DOs

1. When placing the bags at the top thighs in a supine BEING pose, be sure the knees are either on the same plane as the hips or no more than 1 inch above.
2. When grounding the lower back in a prone BEING pose, place the bag directly across the back perpendicular to the spine, with the short ends of the bag facing each hip.
3. Any time you use the bag to ground the shoulders in a supine BEING pose, the back of the outer shoulders should not be more than an inch off the floor.

SANDBAG DON'Ts

Never place the bags directly on the knees unless you are following a particular therapeutic practice to encourage a specific result that you fully understand. The weight of a sandbag on the knees in some straight-legged seated positions with additional prop support can help to stretch tight ligaments. But you must know exactly how to do this and why you are doing it. People will place a 10-pound sandbag just about anywhere, thinking it will help. This will not help when used unwisely.

In general, be mindful of how and why you use sandbags around joints.

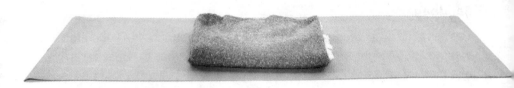

Meditation Pad/Zafu

A meditation pad supports a lift of the spine while in a seated position. Some practitioners use a zafu (from the Japanese word for "round cushion"). Will your meditation be better while sitting on a zafu or pad? That depends. My first meditation teacher taught me how to calm my mind while sitting on a street bench with traffic bustling around me. Would sitting on a zafu have made it better? I have no idea. Some people, however, choose to use one because of a feeling or discipline they've assigned to the object, as some also do with yoga mats. Can we have an active asana (posture) practice without a mat? Absolutely. Do we care for our yoga mats as though they were real estate? Some of us do. In the end, the basic value of having a meditation zafu or a meditation pad made from folding a blanket is that it lifts the pelvis higher than the legs, which makes sitting upright easier.

HOW TO USE: Sit on it, and practice being still. That's it.

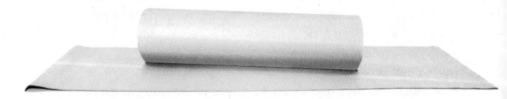

Foam Roller

Two words: Love it! Foam rollers come in several sizes and degrees of density and help to massage large muscle groups and fascia, the fibrous tissue that covers the muscles. Using a roller is almost like getting a massage, except you don't have to pay for it, remove your clothes, or get greased with oil. It does a great job of breaking up lactic acid, and you're in control of the pressure and duration. Of course, rolling on a tennis ball also does the trick, but the body rollers are far superior because of their size, shape, and density. Sometimes I like to start a class, a private session, or my own practice with the foam roller to encourage oxygen and blood flow to muscles. Other times I might end with the roller. It all depends on what I'm trying to support in the practice.

HOW TO USE: Just roll your body across it. You can roll across the front, back, and sides of the body. Roll slowly. If you rip through this action at lightning speed, you won't feel or realize its effects.

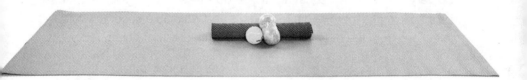

Tennis Ball

As mentioned above, if you don't have a foam roller, a tennis ball can be an adequate and inexpensive replacement. What's effective about using tennis balls is that they can really work the small muscle groups.

HOW TO USE: Roll the ball with the soles of your feet — wonderful for those suffering from plantar fasciitis, a symptom of tight tendons in the soles. You can use it for the spine as well, basically like the foam roller, but since the ball's surface isn't nearly as large as the roller's, be careful when using it near the spinal column. Don't push it directly against the spine; just roll it on either side. You can also tape two tennis balls together so that they can roll in tandem up and down each side of the spinal column.

Eye Pillow

Choosing an eye pillow is sort of like the story "Goldilocks and the Three Bears." You may like an eye pillow that covers the entire forehead. Or perhaps you want one that covers only the eye lids and the bridge of the nose. Or perhaps you want one that falls somewhere in between. Why not have a collection of all sizes so that you can use them as you wish? If you are handy with a sewing machine, you can make these yourself. Eye pillows are typically filled with a mixture of flax seeds, lavender buds, and peppermint and/or chamomile leaves. The smell of this mixture can be very calming and soothing. If you do make any for yourself, please be sure to make them with a removable and washable cover to avoid eye infections from the dirt and dust that accumulate from continued use.

HOW TO USE: I consider eye pillows wonderful little gifts from yoga heaven. They can be used to block out the light, give a little bit of weight to the forehead or the palm of your hands, or provide a cool support under the back of your neck. They support a meaningful turning inward.

GOING DEEPER: THE RIGHTNESS OF PRACTICE

Much of an intelligent and creative yoga practice is getting yourself to see the wisdom of what you are doing and why. It is up to you to bring the kind of awareness to your practice that will clarify what you choose in order to make your practice meaningful. You will never know what comes from your practice if you don't practice with devotion, concentration, and faith.

Learning a Skill

The right prop support can teach a skill necessary for experiencing a balanced approach for doing, being in, and breathing in a yoga pose. Some solutions for addressing difficulties in a pose may often be found in other poses that require less. And solutions will always include a soft breath and a calm mind — in essence, a yielding body and mind. Yoga poses require not only strength, stability, flexibility, and mobility but also skills such as proprioception (the unconscious perception of movement and spatial orientation arising from stimuli within the body itself), somatic movement (movement that relies on an awareness, desire, and ability to become more self-determining; *somatic* refers to your ability to sense the processes going on "within" you), and a mind that doesn't react to its own fluctuations. If one or more of these skills are significantly impaired, the benefits are that much harder to achieve. For instance, let's use a simple back bend as an example.

Back bends require the chest muscles to stretch, the mid and upper back muscles to contract, shoulder mobility, and the fibrous tissue between the mid and upper back vertebrae to move forward. Muscles that are too tight and joints that are too stiff end up relying on help from other areas of the body that aren't meant to play a significant role in the pose. In a classic back-bending pose, this can put strain on the lower segment of the spine and disrupt proper rotation of the shoulder joints. These imbalances, if not addressed, make it difficult to open and lift the chest with strong back body support, a skill necessary for a safe back bend. Therefore, safe and enjoyable back bends are often inaccessible to many students.

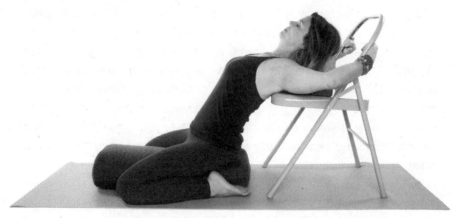

The photo above demonstrates a simple chair-supported Ustrasana (Camel Pose). This variation (see page 51) allows you to breathe and soften in the pose and explore areas that otherwise would not safely be available in a back bend. With the chair, you can investigate the skill necessary to stretch and contract the muscles needed to support a healthy back bend without additional load on the lower back. Benefits abound.

Acceptance — Meet Yourself Where You Are

I am reminded of a workshop I taught for yoga teachers at a body/mind conference. We covered a lot of pose breakdowns, which is always rewarding. Troubleshooting solutions for different body types is a little like being in a lab. You never know how one insight will lead to another, so it is important to be open to the process. The only formula I know for this is meeting students where they are. I practice this acceptance on the mat. It's not always easy, but it is always inspiring.

Throughout my travels, I've had the privilege of working with yoga instructors and students from all over North America and Canada. My experience in general is that too many practitioners feel bad when they run across a yoga pose they cannot execute well. What's worse, I have perceived embarrassment and almost shame. I hear rumblings like, "My shoulders aren't as flexible as Eric's." Or teachers share their concern when they aren't as mobile as some of their students. My advice: welcome acceptance.

NEWS FLASH: There may be poses that you will never be able to practice well without accepting additional support. Or you may come to the realization that some poses aren't right for your body type. Don't feel defeated. Instead, consider this as a giving moment to embrace what is present. Adjust to the utter kindness of accepting support and letting go into what's happening now. Strategic yoga prop support can help you learn how to safely and efficiently leverage your strengths, play with weaknesses, and explore them with a soft breath and calm mind. Sweet relief.

When you step onto your mat, do you ask, "How can I grow today?" or "How can I be more of myself today?" The time on our mat can be used to address these deep questions by recognizing and attending to our individual needs at the moment. Meeting ourselves where we are shines a light on what may be a missing ingredient in many yoga practices: acceptance and mindfulness of what is happening now. Learning how to efficiently use the body and breath as resources to focus, grow, or transform can bring attention to opening and integrating the Light that lives within.

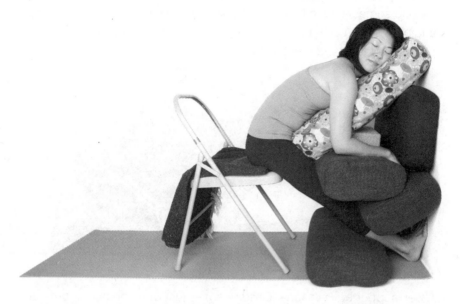

I have a history of tight hamstrings and calves and a tight mid and upper back. This makes forward bends of all kinds my least favorite poses. The variation of Paschimottanasana (Seated Forward Bend Pose) shown in the photo above (and explained on page 91) offers the kind of support needed to move gently into the stretch of my tight legs and back. Yes, it's a lot of support, but I'm not too proud to accept it. Over the years of my practicing this variation from time to time, it has helped me to make great leaps in my forward bending. It has improved my flexibility, and more important, it has taught me how to be more patient in a pose that I previously considered to be my nemesis.

Make It Calmer

Support also comes in the form of feeling that you are so well taken care of that you can completely surrender. Ahhh — nothing quite like it. The body and mind may require a level of healing in a yoga pose that can be offered only when properly supported.

Tom has had a couple of bad bouts with his lower back giving out. One evening he walked into my house for a casual dinner party I was hosting for friends. I watched him walk with a strong lean to one side, like a crab walking on the ocean's uneven sandy bottom. After a visit to the doctor and some yoga therapy, his back healed. But there's nothing more satisfying to someone who has been dealing with back pain than to voice an audible "ahhh" when put into a supported yoga pose that provides both physical release and mental relief.

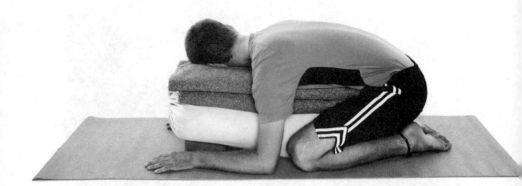

A well-supported Balasana (Child Pose) — just what the doctor ordered.

STRATEGIC PROP PLACEMENT

Pose Alignment and Misalignment

Much of the time we don't know what we are doing while we are doing it, even on the yoga mat. All kinds of misalignments occur without awareness, because habits have deep roots that are invisible to us — that's why they are called habits. Yoga props help us highlight those common and repeated misalignments by preventing us from overworking mobile areas or by stabilizing and stretching underworked ones.

Bringing the Pose to You

Prop support is an important element to having a safe and effective Yapana practice. If the support is inaccurate and does not meet your needs, the benefits of the pose are compromised. There are two ways to bring the pose to you: reducing the reach and broadening the base (see page 33). Each of these addresses our flexibility and/or mobility challenges. And they both take strain away from the joints and an unnecessary load on one or more segments of the spine. Both should encourage space and traction, or extension and contraction, when required.

Awakening Consciousness

A yoga prop can awaken dormant areas of the body, thereby allowing the practitioner to experience a part of the pose that was previously un-reachable. If inflexibility is the only reason a part of a pose has been avoided, the right prop support will build awareness of an unvisited area of the body and create a pathway to improved flexibility.

Quieting Overworked Areas

It's common to overwork yoga poses. Props help all practitioners (includ-ing the most advanced) gain sensitivity by turning off the larger muscle groups and turning on the smaller ones. Yoga props provide support for the overworked areas of the body and allow the mind to relax and both the body and the mind to more profoundly receive the benefits of the practice.

Whether you seek to awaken consciousness or quiet overworked areas, props provide feedback, allowing you to make adjustments in both the body and the mind.

Experiencing the Sweet Sensation

There's nothing wrong with a prop-supported yoga pose that just makes you feel "ahhh." In fact, this is the start of getting in touch with the "rest and digest" system at the center of this practice and the goal in all of the BEING poses.

Waiting

You may set yourself up in a prop-supported pose and not feel the level of stretch you typically feel when practicing the pose without support. What you need to know is sometimes you have to let the pose "bake" for a while. You have to wait. When a pose is well supported, which is different from it being too supported, you may not feel anything, because you are used to the immediate feedback you receive from larger muscle groups firing. Give yourself a bit of time, perhaps a minute or so, to allow the smaller muscles to begin to fire and the sensations to begin to percolate. On the basis of your experience, you can adjust accordingly.

Overpropping Is Overrated

Be careful not to overprop the poses. Recognize the architecture and trajectory of the pose to maintain safe alignment skills and intelligent support that promotes smooth and steady breath and a calm mind. The body should be able to move, if necessary, while in the pose. Notice if the body is moving in relation to the breath — is movement concentrated in one area, or is no movement present? Too many props result in falling into or pushing away from the support. There is a better way.

Pose Trajectory — What Are You Trying to Achieve?

Each pose has a certain architecture that determines the classification of the pose, whether it is standing, back bending, twisting, forward bending, side bending, sitting, or inverting. They all have an intention, purpose, and direction and offer different remedies for the body and mind. Maintaining the trajectory of a pose when supporting it with a prop will help you achieve the purpose for practicing it. For instance, if the BEING back bend that you have propped is not bending the back, clearly it can no longer be considered a back bend. That's why sometimes you have to give up something in order to get something else.

Giving Up Something to Get Something Else

You may find that some of the poses don't work for your level of flexibility. *Don't worry.* What is unique about Yapana practice is that you can attend to those inflexible areas by permitting yourself to safely target them even if you have to give up some of the pose. Ask yourself the following questions:

Why are you practicing a forward bend? So that you can stretch your hamstrings, soothe and calm your central nervous system, or both? If you are pushing yourself in the pose because of tight hamstrings but the pose doesn't generate smooth and steady breath and a calm mind, it's not going to calm the nervous system.

Which is more important to you right now? Does stretching your hamstrings have precedence over the cooling effects of a forward bend or vice versa? Either answer is acceptable and valuable. If you need to address your hamstrings, give up the forward bend and safely target the hamstrings in another supported pose that doesn't require you to do a forward bend. If you need to calm your central nervous system, consider practicing a pose that calms your nervous system and doesn't pull on your short hamstrings. Yapana practice can answer your needs and provide you with ways to meet them while supporting you throughout the journey.

Help for Hyperextension

A hyperextended joint is one that moves beyond its natural range of motion. As a result, additional strain is placed on ligaments and tendons, which help to prevent excessive motion. When these tissues are too loose, the joint is insecure, which can lead to injury. Hyperextension also creates misalignment and poor movement habits that can set the stage for arthritis and other serious conditions. A strategically placed yoga prop can teach how to access neighboring muscles, which are needed to prevent further damage.

HYPEREXTENDED KNEES

In normal standing alignment, the leg forms a straight line from ankle to hip, with knees over ankles and hips over knees. If the knee is hyperextended, however, the leg will appear to curve back, with the knee behind an imaginary straight line drawn from ankle to hip. One leg may hyperextend more than the other. Yoga poses cannot shorten overstretched knee ligaments, but choosing the right poses with the proper support can help stabilize the knees by strengthening the neighboring muscles.

Those who hyperextend their knees have difficulty straightening their legs without overstretching. Because none of the BEING poses require standing, there is less impact on the joints. Some BEING poses, however, require straight and firm legs, such as seated forward bends. These poses can overstretch the knee ligaments unless the knees are properly supported. One rule of thumb is to prop the backs of the knees with minimal support. The support acts as a dam and prevents the knees from moving too far back so that they don't load the weight into ligamentous tissue. This is especially helpful in protecting the knees in forward bends. When the torso moves forward, its relationship to gravity introduces force to the legs and spine.

Adding, Reducing, or Filling Space

Those who are less flexible may require more prop height (adding space) in a BEING pose to compensate for their stiffness in the pose. Conversely, hypermobile people, too, may require more prop height (adding space) in order to avoid falling or collapsing.

Those with a general level of flexibility may require less height (reducing space) in a BEING pose if a bolster or block props them up too much.

A BEING pose may require empty space to be filled between the support, a limb, or other body part and the floor so that the body doesn't feel as though it is in pieces or so that the distal (farthest away) part of the limb is not out of alignment with the largest joint. For instance, in a supine twist, the foot of the top leg should be mostly on the same plane as the top hip rather than dangling below it. Use support to fill the spaces between a student's body and the floor so that the body can receive feedback from the support. This helps to bring the floor to the student and prevents rigidity in the pose or falling out of it.

THINGS TO WATCH OUT FOR

- Avoid sharp angles in the body. The lines of the body should be round and soft, especially in the spine. If in a back bend you see the lumbar (lower back) extended and the thorax (middle back) flat (like an L shape), this indicates that all the segments of the spine are not getting equal work and the load of the pose is resting in the lumbar. Ouch!
- Place, replace, and adjust props to bring the pose to the student, not the student to the pose.

- Use enough props so that the "energy flow" of the pose is not falling backward or behind the head in a back bend.
- Avoid collapsing downward at the torso in a forward bend.
- Avoid collecting the energy flow in the neck in a twist.
- Avoid falling behind the head or collapsing in the lumbar spine in an inversion.

SAFE ALIGNMENT SKILLS (SAS) FOR BEING POSES

All movement requires that alignment principles are maintained in order to avoid injuries, and the practice of BEING poses is no exception to that rule. Safe alignment skills must be maintained in all BEING poses.

Foundation

The foundation of any pose is where everything starts. Perhaps you have heard the foundation of a yoga pose compared to the foundation of a house. The comparison is true. If the foundation of the pose is poor, the rest of the posture is affected. In BEING poses, the setup of the pose provides a solid foundation for safely and easily being and breathing in the pose. No exceptions.

- The body should be positioned with safe and secure alignment.
- The yoga props should be supportive, providing opportunities for both stability and flexibility.

Pelvic Positions

There are three pelvic positions:

1. **NEUTRAL:** pelvis level with natural curve in the lumbar (lower spine).
2. **ANTERIOR TILT:** pelvis tilted forward, bringing the tailbone up and back and the pubis forward.
3. **POSTERIOR TILT:** pelvis tilted backward, bringing the tailbone under and the pubis up.

In any given BEING pose, depending upon the architecture, one of the above positions may be required. Generally, a back bend requires a posterior-tilted pelvis, a forward bend requires an anterior-tilted pelvis, and inversions, twists, and poses that are practiced supine or prone require a neutral pelvis.

Hip Hinge

Many people bend at the hips and waist at the same time when moving forward from an upright (standing or seated) position. Such biomechanics create a considerable strain on the lumbar. When bending forward from either a standing or a seated position, we want to encourage bending at the hips while maintaining a neutral spine and pelvis. A proper hip hinge is necessary in all forward bending and requires two-thirds extension into the pose prior to flexion.

Shoulder Stability/Mobility

The shoulder is a very complicated part of the human body. It is entirely dependent on nonbony connections for integrity. Yoga poses that help both to create stability and to free up mobility are key to injury prevention and good posture. Healthy function of the shoulder is a delicate balance of strength, flexibility, core stability, and alignment.

SHOULDER MOBILITY

Some day-to-day activities, from sitting for long hours at the computer to driving in the car, keep the head in a forward position, which forces the shoulders to be rounded and the chest to sink. Over time this poor postural habit will reduce shoulder mobility (the ability to have free range of motion in the shoulder), and as a result, chronic tension in the neck and upper back will develop. Some BEING poses require shoulder mobility. Safe alignment is paramount to maintain this mobility. Follow these simple rules:

- Drop the shoulders away from the ears.
- When stretching the arms overhead, draw the upper arm bones into the shoulder sockets and keep the shoulder blades firm against the back. This will stabilize the shoulders and enhance movement of the upper extremity when the shoulder goes through its range of motion.

Lightening the Load

There are times when you may need to "lighten the load" in any one of the BEING poses in order to transfer weight equally through the position and maintain SAS. The following are two ways to lighten the load.

BROADENING THE BASE

Broadening the base is needed when more space is required to better access flexibility and SAS. For instance, in Paschimottanasana (Seated Forward Bend Pose), you might require more room in your hips in order to manage short hamstrings, which tend to pull the pelvis under in this seated position. Widening the legs a bit can give more space to the hips and will also help with the hip hinge SAS.

REDUCING THE REACH

Reducing the reach of a pose, whether it is in the lower or upper body, helps to bring the pose to the student rather than the student to the pose, without compromising the general trajectory of the pose. For instance, in Paschimottanasana (Seated Forward Bend Pose), you might require more length in the lower back in order to prevent flexing (rounding) it. Bringing support closer or higher, whether it involves placing a chair or a bolster in front of you or sitting on support to raise the pelvis, reduces the reach in the pose.

CHAPTER 3

AWAKENING: BACK BENDS

The floor beneath you will prevent you from doing anything other than facing yourself, and so it goes with all BEING poses.

A yoga back bend should have these three things: a stable structure, soft lines to its shape, and ample open space. In theory, it should also rival the suspension of the Brooklyn Bridge.

Some students turn away from or fear back bends (the same is true of inversions). Consider these commonly used phrases: "It was a real back bender" and "I bent over backward for her." Each has its own negative connotation, but more important, they both convey that back bending is unpleasant. The truth is, back bending is unpleasant when done incorrectly, unsafely, and without an understanding of the biomechanics. Prone back bends are different from supine back bends. The great thing about practicing back bends restoratively is that they can be targeted to address your specific challenges without overloading any one segment of the spine. You can gain spinal flexibility without putting undue stress on the disks. When practiced safely, however, weight-bearing back bends are equally important because they promote strong and healthy bones.

A range of emotions may surface while you're practicing BEING back bends, but these poses are not to be forced. Rather, when supported they can be an opportunity to evoke a deep acceptance in matters of the heart or to encourage simply receiving the moment as it arises with whatever it may bring. BEING back-bend poses encourage a slow and steady opening in the chest and front body. Supported relaxing back bends may appear as if not much is going on compared to DOING back-bend poses; however, looks are deceiving. Back bends are the most energetic of the BEING poses. They stretch small spinal muscle groups over time, but because they do not require any effort at all, they are also relaxing — involving just breathing, feeling, and sensing.

General Contraindications for Back Bends

- Serious back, neck, shoulder, or knee injury — consult a qualified yoga therapist
- Insomnia
- Migraine
- Recent abdominal or chest surgery

General Benefits of Back Bends

- Keep spine flexible
- Massage and stimulate organs
- Aid digestion
- Release and repattern hyperkyphosis
- Ease depression — proceed slowly and with caution
- Improve asthma — proceed slowly and with caution

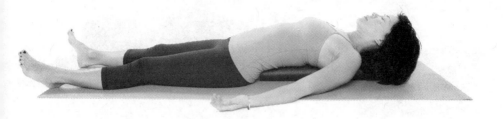

BASIC MATSYASANA (FISH POSE)

How to Move into Basic Matsyasana

1. Roll a thin yoga mat from the short side.
2. Place the short end of the mat up against the spine, either at the lower back or at the base of the back ribs. Be sure to support the head.
3. Stretch out the legs and arms.
4. Breathe and relax.

How to Come out of Basic Matsyasana

1. Release the arms if they are stretched overhead.
2. Bend the knees, and set the feet onto the floor.
3. Draw the left arm in to the chest.
4. Push off with the feet, and roll to the right side.
5. Pause.
6. Prepare for what's next.

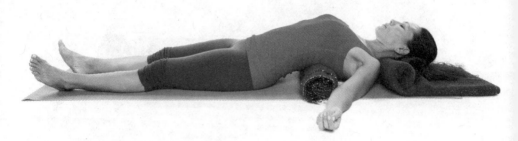

MATSYASANA, VAR. 1 (FISH POSE, VAR. 1)

How to Move into Matsyasana, Var. 1

In variation 1 of Matsyasana, the blankets are rolled to support the level of opening you wish to receive in the chest and neck.

1. Position two long-rolled blankets behind you and across the mat, approximately 1 foot away from each other.
2. Sit in front of the first blanket with your knees bent. Using your hands for support, lie back until the shoulder blades rest across that blanket, the arms fit between the two blankets, and the neck or head is supported on the second blanket.
3. Stretch the legs out, and keep them hip-width distance apart.
4. Allow the arms to relax with the palms turned upward.
5. Relax the front bottom ribs.
6. Breathe and relax.

How to Come out of Matsyasana, Var. 1

Follow the basic pose instructions (page 38).

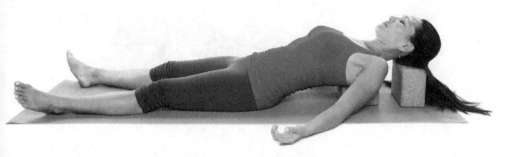

MATSYASANA, VAR. 2 (FISH POSE, VAR. 2)

How to Move into Matsyasana, Var. 2

Two blocks are used in variation 2 of Matsyasana to provide solid support for the mid and upper back. The blocks can be laid flat, placed on edge, or stood on end. Laying the block flat and placing it at the mid back provides superficial support against the muscles, while placing it on edge offers more feedback against the spinal ligaments of the mid back. Standing it on end provides the most stimulation.

1. Position two yoga blocks at the top of the yoga mat — one laid flat and the other placed on edge.
2. With your knees bent, sit in front of the first block, and using your hands for support, lie back until the shoulder blades rest across the block and the head rests on the other block.
3. Stretch the legs out, and keep them hip-width distance apart.
4. Allow the arms to relax with the palms turned upward.
5. Relax the front bottom ribs.
6. Breathe and relax.

How to Come out of Matsyasana, Var. 2

Follow the basic pose instructions (page 38).

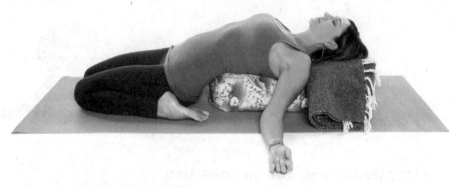

BASIC SUPTA VIRASANA (RECLINING HERO POSE)

Supta Virasana is a back bend that gives a big stretch to the front thigh muscles (quadriceps), knees, and ankles. The basic version of this pose is not for everyone, because it extends the lower back. This is a pose that can be worked up to once the quadriceps are flexible and you have had considerable experience with back bends. However, as an alternative you can increase the angle (reduce the reach) by building up the support so that the pose comes to you instead of requiring you to get into it the basic way. The short end of the bolster can be placed right up against the lower back or against the lower back ribs, depending on whether you prefer the support at the lower back or whether you feel compressed in that position and instead require the lift at the ribs.

How to Move into Basic Supta Virasana

1. Position a bolster on the mat in a parallel orientation, and lay a long-folded blanket across the top end of the bolster.
2. Kneel in front of the bolster with your back facing it, and use the hands to stretch the calf muscles away from the knees and toward the heels.
3. Drop the hips to sit on the floor with the hips between your two feet.
4. Place the hands on the feet to use the arms as leverage to lift the chest and safely lie back on the bolster, resting the head on the blanket.
5. Lift and broaden the chest.
6. Breathe and relax.

How to Come out of Basic Supta Virasana

1. Gently tuck the chin.
2. Push the hands against the feet or the floor to use as leverage to lift up and out of the pose.
3. Pause.
4. Prepare for what's next.

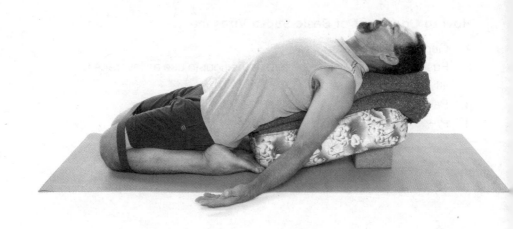

SUPTA VIRASANA, VAR. 1 (RECLINING HERO POSE, VAR. 1)

Try this variation if you need a little more relief in the lower back. Notice how the top end of the bolster is elevated with a block, and two double-folded blankets are stacked on top, with their short ends stair-stepped by approximately 1 inch, to bring further height (reduce the reach) to the student and to better support the back.

How to Move into Supta Virasana, Var. 1

1. Follow the basic pose instructions (page 41) with the modified prop placement.
2. Breathe and relax.

How to Come out of Supta Virasana, Var. 1

Follow the basic pose instructions (page 41).

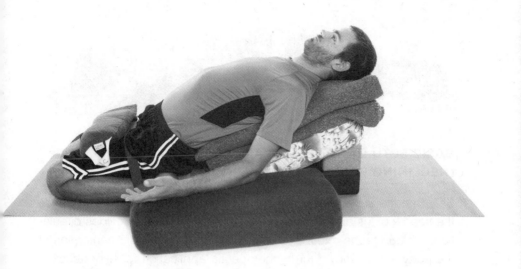

SUPTA VIRASANA, VAR. 2 (RECLINING HERO POSE, VAR. 2)

In variation 2 of Supta Virasana, the pose is considerably elevated in order to meet flexibility challenges. Now the bolster is elevated with two blocks in addition to the further height of the stacked, double-folded blankets. A bolster is also placed on each side of the body to support the arms.

How to Move into Supta Virasana, Var. 2

1. Follow the basic pose instructions (page 40) with the modified prop placement.
2. Breathe and relax.

How to Come out of Supta Virasana, Var. 2

Follow the basic pose instructions (page 41).

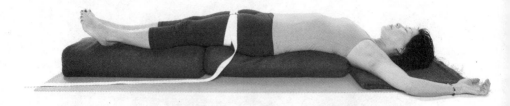

BASIC SETU BANDHA SARVANGASANA
(RECLINING BRIDGE POSE)

Setu Bandha Sarvangasana is a back bend that keeps the heart above the head, so it is also considered a soft inversion that provides circulation of blood to the chest and neck. It lengthens the front center line of the body and is known for its therapeutic application for hypertension. A belt is fastened around the top thighs to keep them from separating while in the pose.

How to Move into Basic Setu Bandha Sarvangasana

1. Prepare the setup by lining up the short ends of two bolsters to make a "bed."
2. Sit on the bolsters with the knees bent, and fasten a belt around the thighs.
3. With the support of your hands and feet, slide back until your upper back, shoulders, and head are resting on the floor.
4. Place your arms in a goalpost position, being sure to keep the backs of the shoulders flat on the ground.
5. Relax the front ribs.
6. Breathe and relax.

How to Come out of Basic Setu Bandha Sarvangasana

1. Release the tension of the belt.
2. Bend the knees, and place the feet on the ground along each side of the bolster.
3. Push off with the feet to slide the body back and off the support until the pelvis and lower back rest on the floor.
4. Draw the knees in to the chest, and roll to the side.
5. Pause.
6. Prepare for what's next.

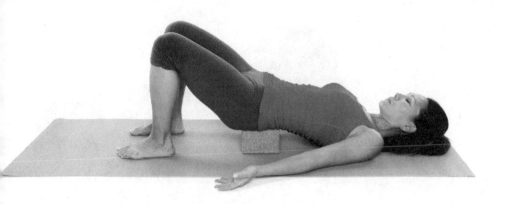

SETU BANDHA SARVANGASANA, VAR. 1
(RECLINING BRIDGE POSE, VAR. 1)

For more lift in the pelvis, variations 1–3 of Setu Bandha Sarvangasana act as stronger inversions, with variations 2 and 3 offering the greatest elevation. The blocks help to stabilize the lower back and sacrum, making them a good choice for those challenged with sacroiliac (SI) joint dysfunction, if stabilization is needed. The SI joint is the connection between the spine and the pelvis. Too much or not enough movement in the joint results in inflammation. It supports the spine by providing stability and acts as a shock absorber for forces to the lower extremities.

How to Move into Setu Bandha Sarvangasana, Var. 1

1. Lie back with the knees bent.
2. Lift the hips, and lay a block flat underneath the tailbone and sacrum. Lower the hips to rest on the block.
3. Relax the arms alongside the body with the hands positioned approximately 6 inches away from the hips and the palms turned up.
4. Relax the shoulders and head.
5. Relax the front ribs.
6. Breathe and relax.

How to Come out of Setu Bandha Sarvangasana, Var. 1

1. Lift the hips, remove the block, and return the body to the ground, keeping the knees bent.
2. Pause.
3. Prepare for what's next.

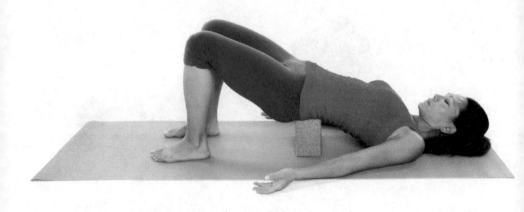

SETU BANDHA SARVANGASANA, VAR. 2
(RECLINING BRIDGE POSE, VAR. 2)

How to Move into Setu Bandha Sarvangasana, Var. 2

1. Follow the pose instructions for variation 1 (page 45), but place the block on edge.
2. Breathe and relax.

How to Come out of Setu Bandha Sarvangasana, Var. 2

Follow the pose instructions for variation 1 (page 45).

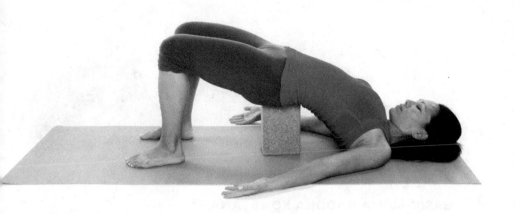

SETU BANDHA SARVANGASANA, VAR. 3
(RECLINING BRIDGE POSE, VAR. 3)

You can play with the height in Setu Bandha Sarvangasana. In variation 3, the block is placed on end. But you might decide to explore even more height than is shown in the photo above by laying a block flat and stacking another block on top, placing it on edge. Explore as you wish, but remember to keep both of the shoulders on the floor no matter how much your pelvis is elevated.

How to Move into Setu Bandha Sarvangasana, Var. 3

1. Follow the pose instructions for variation 1 (page 45) with modified prop placement.
2. Breathe and relax.

How to Come out of Setu Bandha Sarvangasana, Var. 3

Follow the pose instructions for variation 1 (page 45).

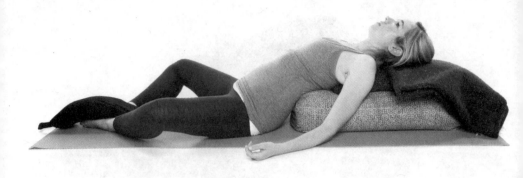

BASIC SUPTA BADDHA KONASANA (RECLINING BOUND ANGLE POSE)

Supta Baddha Konasana is a wonderful pose for the legs and hips. Be sure to support the upper legs if they are above hip level. This way there will not be an uneven load on the hips. The support provides good feedback for the legs to relax. Just as in Supta Virasana (Reclining Hero Pose), the support at the back may be placed directly underneath the lower back or underneath the back ribs. This is a pose that everyone can practice, and I haven't met anyone who hasn't enjoyed being in it. Like all of the poses, it only needs to meet you where you are.

How to Move into Basic Supta Baddha Konasana

1. Position a bolster on your mat in a parallel orientation and one or two single-folded blankets at the top end of the bolster.
2. Sit in front of the short end of the bolster, and bring the soles of the feet together so that the knees fall to the sides.
3. For additional "grounding," place a 10-pound sandbag on the feet.
4. Using your hands for support, gently lie back onto the support.
5. Allow the lower body to relax and sink into the floor and the upper body to open.
6. Breathe and relax.

How to Come out of Basic Supta Baddha Konasana

1. Gently tuck the chin.
2. Use the hands as leverage against the floor to lift up and out of the pose.

3. Slide one foot out to the side, and then straighten the leg, followed by the other foot and leg.
4. Pause with the legs straight, and sit upright.
5. Prepare for what's next.

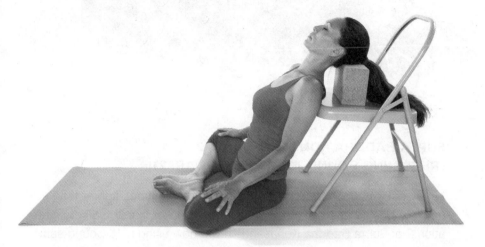

SUPTA BADDHA KONASANA, VAR. 1
(RECLINING BOUND ANGLE POSE, VAR. 1)

Variation 1 of Supta Baddha Konasana is a lovely way to get the opening in the mid back and legs without having to be in a fully reclined position.

How to Move into Supta Baddha Konasana, Var. 1

1. Position a chair on the yoga mat with a yoga block on the seat.
2. Sit in front of the chair, and bring the soles of the feet together so that the knees fall to the sides.
3. Using the hands for support, lift the chest while leaning back to rest the bottom of the shoulder blades against the front lip of the chair seat.
4. Rest your hands on your legs and your head on the block.
5. Sink the lower body into the floor, and relax the front ribs.
6. Breathe and relax.

How to Come out of Supta Baddha Konasana, Var. 1

Follow the basic pose instructions (page 48).

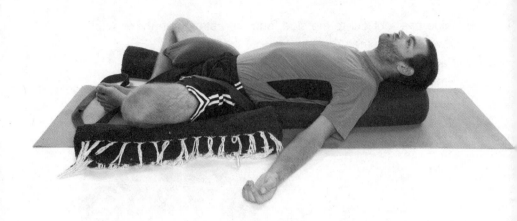

SUPTA BADDHA KONASANA, VAR. 2
(RECLINING BOUND ANGLE POSE, VAR. 2)

Imbalances happen in all of us. One shoulder or hip is tighter than the other, or one segment of the spine is much weaker than the others. Variation 2 of Supta Baddha Konasana shows how using a 10-pound sandbag on the tighter leg can help to even out flexibility challenges. A yoga belt is fastened around the lower back, running down across the inner legs, and then around the outer feet in order to help stabilize the pelvis as the pose stretches out the lower body. And this variation shows the short end of the bolster positioned right underneath the lower back and without any blanket support on top of it. Long-rolled blankets are placed underneath the upper thighs and shins to support the legs in the stretch.

How to Move into Supta Baddha Konasana, Var. 2

1. Follow the basic pose instructions (page 48) with modified prop placement.
2. Breathe and relax.

How to Come out of Supta Baddha Konasana, Var. 2

Follow the basic pose instructions (page 48).

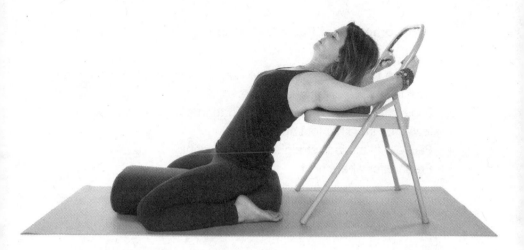

BASIC USTRASANA (CAMEL POSE)

The Basic Ustrasana back bend is a good alternative for opening the chest in a seated position with a leg stretch similar to the one done in classic Camel Pose, kneeling on the knees. Of course, you can change the leg position to your preference. This is a combination of Basic Virasana (Hero Pose) in the lower body and Supta Baddha Konasana, Var. 1 (Reclining Bound Angle Pose, Var. 1) in the upper body. You can change the upper body and lower body positions to meet any criterion or creative urge.

How to Move into Basic Ustrasana

1. Position a sturdy chair on the mat. Place a block on the seat, parallel to the rung on the seat back, and a bolster in front of the chair.
2. Straddle the bolster with your legs folded behind you and your back facing the chair.
3. Using the hands for support, lift the chest while leaning back to rest the bottom of the shoulder blades against the front lip of the chair and your head on the block. If necessary, adjust the height of the block so the head can rest comfortably on it.
4. Rest your hands on your thighs, or hold on to the back of the chair for a deeper chest and shoulder stretch.
5. Relax the front ribs.
6. Breathe and relax.

How to Come out of Basic Ustrasana

1. Gently tuck the chin.
2. Release the arms, and use the hands as leverage against the floor to lift up and out of the pose.
3. Slide one foot out to the side, and then straighten the leg, followed by the other foot and leg.
4. Pause with the legs straight, and sit upright.
5. Prepare for what's next.

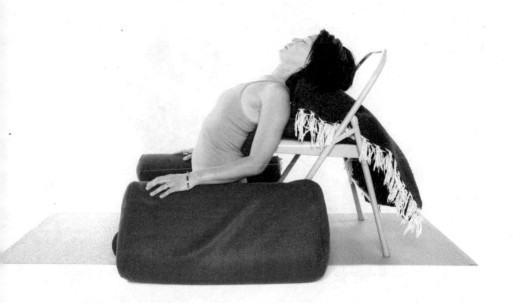

USTRASANA, VAR. 1 (CAMEL POSE, VAR. 1)

Variation 1 of Ustrasana offers additional lift in the mid back for those who may require it. If you don't feel the chest "popping" in Basic Ustrasana (without the front ribs being aggressively pushed forward), this modification will provide it. Simply drape a long-folded blanket over the front lip of the chair; on top of that, near the center of the chair seat, place a block on edge, parallel to the rung on the seat back; and finally place a long-folded blanket on top of the block, to support the back of the head. Positioning two bolsters on either side of the hips creates perfect armrests.

How to Move into Ustrasana, Var. 1

Follow the basic pose instructions (page 51) with modified prop placement but without extending the arms, instead resting them on the bolsters.

How to Come out of Ustrasana, Var. 1

Follow the basic pose instructions (page 52).

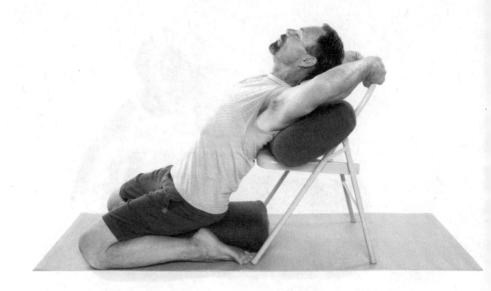

USTRASANA, VAR. 2 (CAMEL POSE, VAR. 2)

For less of a mid and upper back bend in Ustrasana, a bolster is placed on the chair seat to meet flexibility challenges (reduce the reach). The angle of the bolster supports the back of the shoulders and the shoulder blades. This allows tight shoulders to stretch without compromising safe alignment.

How to Move into Ustrasana, Var. 2

Follow the basic pose instructions (page 51) with modified prop placement.

How to Come out of Ustrasana, Var. 2

Follow the basic pose instructions (page 52).

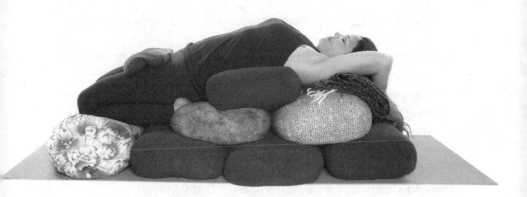

BASIC VIPARITA DANDASANA
(INVERTED TWO-LEGGED STAFF POSE)

If you have many bolsters, the Viparita Dandasana back bend provides ample support to all segments of the spine. Be sure to follow the instructions for coming out of this pose. Curling up out of it or rolling to one side puts too much load on the back. Instead, you'll slide your way out head first and enjoy every minute of it.

How to Move into Basic Viparita Dandasana

1. Position three bolsters next to one another on the mat in a perpendicular orientation.
2. Stack two more bolsters, centered on top of the first three.
3. Stack one more bolster on top, centered, so the shape looks similar to a pyramid.
4. On the middle layer of bolsters, position a meditation pad or double-folded blanket along the outer edge of the bolster where the head will rest. Then add a fourth bolster to the first layer, at the end of the mat where the legs will go.
5. Using your hands for support, kneel on the fourth bolster of the bottom layer. Use your hands to stretch the calf muscles away from the knees and toward the heels. Drop the hips to sit on the edge of the nearest bolster of the middle layer.
6. Lean back so the lower and mid back are supported by the top center bolster and the neck waterfalls off the back edge of the

middle-layer bolster where you've placed the double-folded blanket. Knees should rest on the fourth bolster.

7. Stretch the arms overhead, shoulder distance apart, with the palms facing each other.

8. Bend the elbows and tuck the palms, now facing downward, behind the bolster beneath your head, and keep the elbows shoulder distance apart.

9. Breathe and relax.

How to Come out of Basic Viparita Dandasana

1. Release the arms from overhead.
2. Place your hands against the bottom layer of bolsters.
3. Slide one foot out to the side, and then straighten the leg, followed by the other foot and leg.
4. Tuck your chin, and with control, push with your hands and feet to slowly slide off the support in the direction of your head, until your lower back and hips touch the floor and your lower legs rest on the support.
5. Pause.
6. Prepare for what's next.

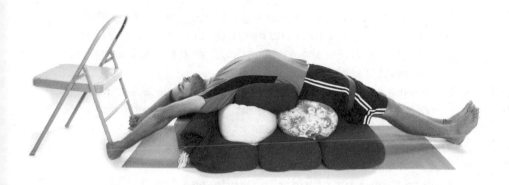

VIPARITA DANDASANA, VAR. 1
(INVERTED TWO-LEGGED STAFF POSE, VAR. 1)

In variation 1 of Viparita Dandasana, the shoulders are in full flexion behind the head. In variation 2, the shoulders are stretched but you support them for safe alignment by holding on to the legs of a chair placed at the far end of the pyramid of bolsters. Also at the far end, a block has replaced a blanket for the headrest, to increase the height of the head support. To prevent the legs from separating, which can put undue pressure on the lumbar, fasten a belt around the top thighs. This is similar to being stretched on a rack — in a good way! It offers tremendous traction to unfurl any tight spots in the back.

How to Move into Viparita Dandasana, Var. 1

1. Place a chair on the floor a few inches from one end of your mat, with the back of the chair facing the mat. Have a belt nearby.
2. Position three bolsters next to each other on the mat in a perpendicular orientation. At the end of the bolsters close to the chair, where the head will rest, place a block on the floor touching the bolster.
3. Stack two more bolsters, centered on top of the first three.
4. Stack one more bolster on top, centered, so the shape looks similar to a pyramid.
5. Place a rolled blanket on the bolster in the first layer that's closest to the block. This blanket will support the shoulders.
6. Using your hands for support, sit on the edge of the nearest bolster of the middle layer.

7. Fasten a belt around the top thighs to keep the legs together.
8. Lean back so the lower and mid back are supported by the top center bolster, the shoulders are supported by the blanket, and the head is supported by the block.
9. Stretch the arms overhead, shoulder distance apart, with the palms facing each other, and grasp one chair leg with each hand. Push the chair away until the arms are straight.
10. Breathe and relax.

How to Come out of Viparita Dandasana, Var. 1

1. Bend the knees and place the feet on a bolster.
2. Place your hands against the bottom layer of bolsters.
3. Tuck your chin, and with control, push with your hands and feet to slowly slide partially off the bolsters in the direction of your head, until you can push the chair farther away from you.
4. Slide back until your lower back and hips touch the floor and your lower legs rest on the bolsters.
5. Pause.
6. Prepare for what's next.

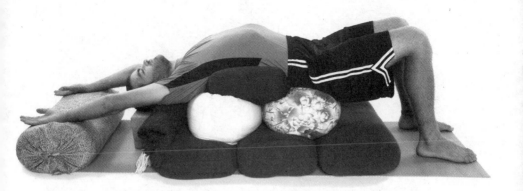

VIPARITA DANDASANA, VAR. 2
(INVERTED TWO-LEGGED STAFF POSE, VAR. 2)

If the extension on the lower back is too much in variation 1 of Viparita
Dandasana, simply bend the knees and place the feet flat on the floor. If
the flexion of the arms is too much in variation 1, the head will drop below
the shoulders and the shoulder joints may impinge. In this case, in addition to supporting the head with a block to keep it on the same plane as
the shoulders, a bolster can be positioned underneath the forearms and
hands to keep the shoulders and head aligned.

How to Move into Viparita Dandasana, Var. 2

1. Follow the variation 1 pose instructions (page 57) with modified
   prop placement.
2. Breathe and relax.

How to Come out of Viparita Dandasana, Var. 2

Follow the variation 1 pose instructions (page 58).

CHAPTER 4

UNWINDING: TWISTS

....

*Yapana BEING twists are calming to the nervous system
and improve vertebral joint flexibility.*

BEING twist poses involve opposing movements; a straight line is maintained in the spine while the pelvis and shoulder girdles stack. They can be practiced as a wringing-out movement, where more emphasis is placed on rotation, or as a spiral movement, with more emphasis on thoracic extension. In either case, torque on the lumbar should be avoided, and thoracic rotation should be the main focus. You can begin your practice with a twist as long as it is followed by a pose that puts the spine in a neutral position, such as Child Pose, Half Knee to Chest Pose, or a forward bend — anything that doesn't rotate or bend the spine right away.

Miraculously, BEING twists seem to untether the knots stored in the back. Many students, after practicing BEING twists, experience the unwinding of accumulated stress. BEING twists are calming to the nervous system and improve vertebral joint flexibility.

General Contraindications for BEING Twists

- Sciatica
- Sacroiliac joint dysfunction
- Herniated disks

- Pregnancy
- Recent abdominal surgery

General Benefits of BEING Twists

- Improve vertebral joint flexibility
- Improve digestion
- Improve circulation by squeezing and soaking the internal organs in blood

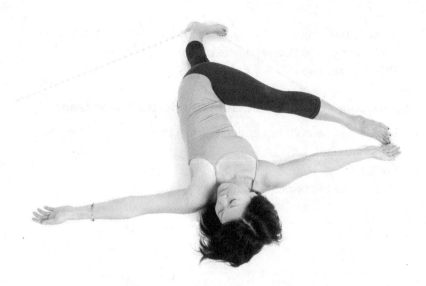

BASIC SUPTA PARIVRTTA TRIKONASANA
(RECLINING REVOLVED TRIANGLE POSE)

Supta Parivrtta Trikonasana is a supine (on the back) take on the classic standing version: Revolved Triangle Pose. This deep twist can be practiced with either a wringing-out or a spiral movement in the thoracic. Play with the two to see which offers you the most opening without disturbing the lower back. Both shoulders must remain on the floor while the hips are stacked, so it's not important that the hand reaching toward the foot of the top leg actually touches it. Just move in that direction.

How to Move into Basic Supta Parivrtta Trikonasana

1. Lie on your right side a few feet from a wall, with your torso perpendicular to the wall, your thighs perpendicular to your torso, and your knees bent at a 90° angle.
2. Stretch the left leg forward and the right leg behind you into a "scissor"-legged position.
3. Slide the torso to the right, reaching the right hand toward the left foot.
4. Straighten the legs, gently pressing the right foot into the wall, while turning the torso open so that the back rests flat on the floor.

5. Make small adjustments to comfortably rest the back of the shoulders on the floor while keeping the hips stacked.
6. Breathe and relax.

How to Come out of Basic Supta Parivrtta Trikonasana

1. Draw both the right leg and left arm in to the body's center, and roll to the right.
2. Pause.
3. Prepare for the opposite side.

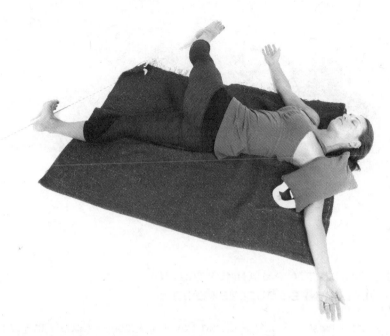

SUPTA PARIVRTTA TRIKONASANA, VAR. 1
(RECLINING REVOLVED TRIANGLE POSE, VAR. 1)

Using a 10-pound sandbag in this variation of Supta Parivrtta Trikona-sana keeps the top shoulder "grounded" and provides that extra bit of opening to a tight chest. Consider using this prop only when the shoulder is already touching the floor. The sandbag should be placed across the front of the shoulder and upper arm that reaches away from the twist but should not be placed on a shoulder that is elevated more than 1 inch above the floor. Avoid placing the bag on the neck or elbow. And remember to keep the hips stacked so that the top hip is not rolling forward of the bottom one. This ensures a steady pelvis for encouraging the twist in the mid back rather than the lower back.

How to Move into Supta Parivrtta Trikonasana, Var. 1

1. Follow the basic pose instructions (page 63) with modified prop placement.
2. Breathe and relax.

How to Come out of Supta Parivrtta Trikonasana, Var. 1

Follow the basic pose instructions (page 64).

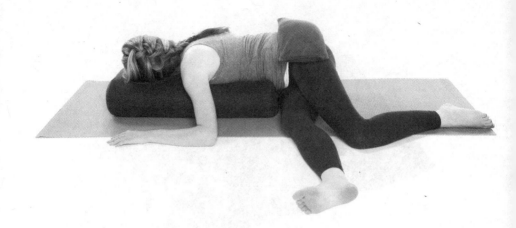

BASIC PARIVRTTA PAVANMUKTASANA (REVOLVED KNEE SQUEEZE POSE)

The relaxing twist in Basic Parivrtta Pavanmuktasana targets the turn of the belly. Because it is a prone (on the belly) twist, the height of the support should allow for the hips and shoulders to be on the same plane. Also, keep the elbows and shoulders on the same plane. First, draw the shoulders down and away from the ears so that they aren't hiking up to the neck. Keeping the arms bent in a 90° position will prevent the shoulders and shoulder blades from lifting. A sandbag placed on the top hip helps to weight the pelvis.

How to Move into Basic Parivrtta Pavanmuktasana

1. Position a bolster on the mat in a parallel orientation.
2. Sit with the right hip against the short side of the bolster, and bend the left leg behind you.
3. Position a sandbag across the top hip.
4. Place your hands on either side of the bolster and push them against the floor, using it as leverage to lift the chest and rotate it and the head to the right side.
5. Lower the torso onto the bolster.
6. Place the arms in a goalpost position.
7. Breathe and relax.

How to Come out of Basic Parivrtta Pavanmuktasana

1. Keep the chin in a neutral position relative to a neutral skull, and turn the head to rest the forehead on the bolster.
2. Place the hands on the floor underneath the shoulders.
3. Push the hands against the floor to straighten the arms and lift the torso away from the bolster.
4. Remove the sandbag.
5. Straighten both legs, and sit upright.
6. Pause.
7. Prepare for the opposite side.

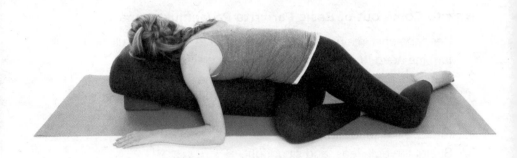

PARIVRTTA PAVANMUKTASANA, VAR. 1
(REVOLVED KNEE SQUEEZE POSE, VAR. 1)

A simple way to keep the shoulders and hips on the same plane in Parivrtta Pavanmuktasana is to elevate the top end of the bolster with a block, as in this variation. Unlike in the basic version, the bottom leg is bent in variation 1, which decreases the stretch of the leg and the lower back.

How to Move into Parivrtta Pavanmuktasana, Var. 1

1. Follow the basic pose instructions (page 66) with modified prop placement.
2. Breathe and relax.

How to Come out of Parivrtta Pavanmuktasana, Var. 1

Follow the basic pose instructions (page 67).

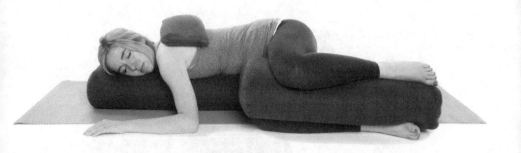

PARIVRTTA PAVANMUKTASANA, VAR. 2
(REVOLVED KNEE SQUEEZE POSE, VAR. 2)

In some cases, tight neck and upper back muscles prevent us from easily turning the head in the opposite direction from the knees. Simply turning the head in the same direction as the knees, along with placing a 10-pound sandbag across the shoulder blades, resolves this. Just that little bit of weight can help relax the muscles so that both shoulders stay on the same plane. This allows the weight of the twist to remain even rather than loading on one side of the body. Placing a bolster between the legs softens the stretch of the top leg and helps to align the hips.

How to Move into Parivrtta Pavanmuktasana, Var. 2

1. Follow the basic pose instructions (page 66) with modified prop placement.
2. Breathe and relax.

How to Come out of Parivrtta Pavanmuktasana, Var. 2

Follow the basic pose instructions (page 67).

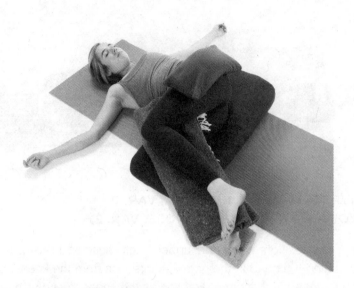

BASIC JATHARA PARIVARTANASANA (STOMACH TURN POSE)

Basic Jathara Parivartanasana is a deep twist that offers a good stretch to the muscles of the top leg and hip because of the elevated pelvis. The basic version has a sandbag placed on the hip to "ground" it and a double-folded blanket between the legs to encourage stacked hips and a gradual release of the lower back. In all variations, align the top hip with the shoulder on that side of the body. Adjust your body accordingly.

How to Move into Basic Jathara Parivartanasana

1. Position a bolster on the floor next to the center of the mat in a perpendicular orientation, place a block approximately 1 foot beyond the top edge of the bolster, and have folded blankets and another block nearby.
2. Lie down on the mat face up with the arms in a T position, the knees bent, and the feet on the floor. Lift the hips and slide the bolster under them, then lower the hips to rest your lower back and pelvis on the bolster.
3. Push your feet against the floor, lift the hips again, and scoot them to the far left of the bolster.

4. Place a double-folded blanket between the legs, and as you lower the knees to the right, stack your feet and rest them on the block.
5. Place a sandbag on the top hip.
6. Breathe and relax.

How to Come out of Basic Jathara Parivartanasana

1. Draw the top knee in to the chest, keeping it close to the torso as you move.
2. Draw the opposite knee in to the chest.
3. When both knees are pulled in toward the chest, place the feet on the floor beyond the bolster.
4. Rest the pelvis and lower back on the center of the bolster.
5. Pause.
6. Prepare for the opposite side.

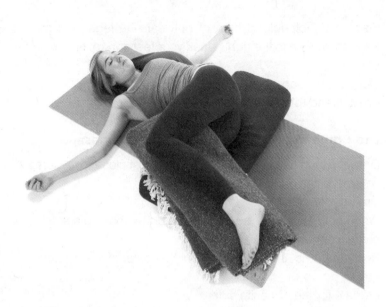

JATHARA PARIVARTANASANA, VAR. 1
(STOMACH TURN POSE, VAR. 1)

Remember, all twists require both shoulders to be resting on the floor to promote a well-balanced rotation in the spine and prevent overloading on one side of the body. If your back muscles are tight, the shoulder farther from the knees will likely lift away from the floor. A sandbag placed on this shoulder encourages it to "ground" and gently coaches it and the back muscles to relax into gravity. A sandbag should not be placed on a shoulder that is elevated more than 1 inch above the floor.

How to Move into Jathara Parivartanasana, Var. 1

1. Follow the basic pose instructions (page 70) with modified prop placement.
2. Breathe and relax.

How to Come out of Jathara Parivartanasana, Var. 1

Follow the basic pose instructions (page 71).

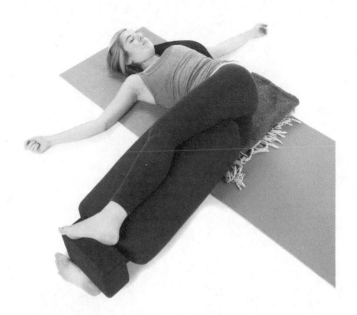

JATHARA PARIVARTANASANA, VAR. 2
(STOMACH TURN POSE, VAR. 2)

Variation 2 of Jathara Parivartanasana offers the strongest of sensations because both legs are straight. Straightening both the legs offers additional stretch to the lower back and legs. A bolster is placed between the legs and a block between the feet to keep the hips stacked, and a sandbag is placed on the shoulder to keep both shoulders on the same plane. The bottom support has been replaced with a double-folded blanket. Breathe into this one!

How to Move into Jathara Parivartanasana, Var. 2

1. Follow the basic pose instructions (page 70) with modified prop placement.
2. Breathe and relax.

How to Come out of Jathara Parivartanasana, Var. 2

Follow the basic pose instructions (page 71).

CHAPTER 5

DECOMPRESSING: INVERSIONS

....

Yapana BEING inversion poses are the easiest way to invert the body with the least amount of work.

Yapana BEING inversion poses are a valuable part of the practice. They are excellent variations of the DOING inversions, have the same benefits, and can be practiced by anyone who is a candidate for inverting.

Going upside down can be scary for some people, even when the pose is well supported. Consider trying the inverted BEING poses that are the least threatening, like "Legs up the Chair," then graduate toward stronger inversions.

General Contraindications for Inversions

- Vertigo
- Glaucoma
- Headache
- Serious heart problems
- Heavy menstruation — first days of heavy bleeding
- Uncontrolled high blood pressure and heart conditions
- Detached retina
- Inflammation of eyes and ears
- Pulled hamstrings — proceed with caution

- Pregnancy — after the first trimester, and even during the first trimester, practice this pose only if you have a regular inversion practice and are comfortable with inverting. Pregnant women are known to become very in tune with their bodies. Follow your instincts.

General Benefits of Inversions
- Help to reverse the effects of gravity
- Relieve tired legs and feet
- Encourage venous return (keep fluids moving toward the heart)
- Refresh the brain with freshly oxygenated blood
- Calm the mind

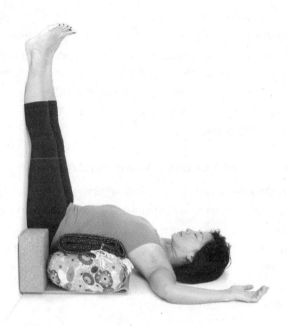

BASIC VIPARITA KARANI
("LEGS UP THE WALL" POSE)

Basic Viparita Karani is an inverted pose that I always practice when traveling. After I settle into my hotel room, I slide my legs up the wall. Many times, I've fallen asleep while in this pose. When you don't have access to your props, just a wall will do.

The shoulders should remain on the floor with the legs straight. You can modify the height of the pelvis from no support at all to a bolster and several blankets for a bigger back bend. You decide what makes sense and supports a smooth and steady breath. In the basic version, the blocks are merely spacers to create distance between the bolster and the wall.

How to Move into Basic Viparita Karani

1. Fold a mat into thirds, and place the long side against the wall.
2. Stand two blocks on end against the wall, lined up with the outer edges of the mat.
3. Lie down on the floor with the pelvis between the two blocks and the legs up the wall.

4. Bend the knees, push the feet against the wall to lift the pelvis, and slide a bolster — and an additional blanket for height, if necessary — underneath the lower and mid back. Allow the pelvis to drop into the space between the bolster and the wall.
5. Bring your arms into a goalpost or a T position.
6. Breathe and relax.

How to Come out of Basic Viparita Karani

1. Bend the knees, pushing the feet against the wall, and slide backward until the pelvis and lower back are resting on the bolster.
2. Pause.
3. Slide back again until the pelvis and lower back are resting on the floor.
4. Pause.
5. Prepare for what's next.

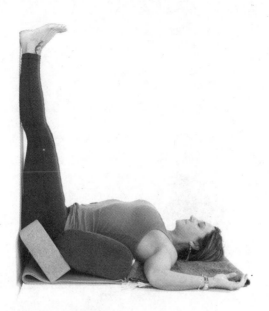

VIPARITA KARANI, VAR. 1
("LEGS UP THE WALL" POSE, VAR. 1)

If your lower back is more flat than arched, variation 1 of Viparita Karani is a simple modification that supports the spine in the architecture of this particular pose. The bolster's elevation by the angled blocks creates an arch in the lower back slightly greater than that of the basic pose. A blanket underneath the shoulders and head may be necessary to fill any space there might be between them and the mat. Keep thinking about how you can bring the pose to the student, not the student to the pose.

How to Move into Viparita Karani, Var. 1

1. Follow the basic pose instructions (page 77) with modified prop placement.
2. Breathe and relax.

How to Come out of Viparita Karani, Var. 1

1. Bend the knees, and place the feet against the wall.
2. Push the feet against the wall to lift the hips off the bolster.
3. Release the pelvis, and lower the back onto the floor.
4. Draw the knees in to the chest, and roll to one side.
5. Pause.
6. Prepare for what's next.

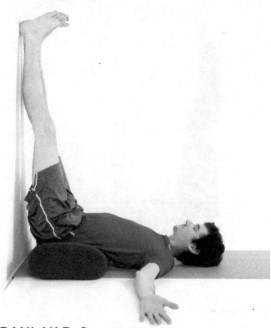

VIPARITA KARANI, VAR. 2
("LEGS UP THE WALL" POSE, VAR. 2)

Tight hamstrings (upper back-leg muscles) will prevent you from bringing the legs flush to the wall in Viparita Karani. In variation 2, the pelvis
and legs do not rest directly against the wall (reducing the reach). If you
attempt this pose with tight hamstrings and a posterior-tilted pelvis, you
will likely not be able to hold yourself on the support without effort. More
important, the lower back is likely to flex, which should be avoided here.

How to Move into Viparita Karani, Var. 2

1. Lie down on the floor, and bring the pelvis either against a wall
   or about 5 to 6 inches away from it, resting the legs up the wall.
2. Bend the knees, push the feet against the wall to lift the pelvis,
   and slide a bolster underneath the pelvis and lower back.
3. Bring your arms into a T position with the palms turned up.
4. Release the weight of your legs into the pelvis and the pelvis into
   the bolster.
5. Breathe and relax.

How to Come out of Viparita Karani, Var. 2

Follow the instructions for variation 1 (page 79).

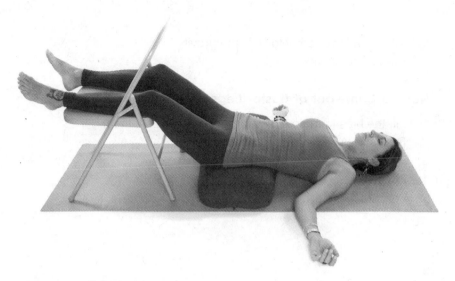

"LEGS UP THE CHAIR" POSE

"Legs up the Chair" Pose is the perfect version of Viparita Karani ("Legs up the Wall" Pose) for someone whose legs keep sliding down the wall because of either very loose ligaments or very tight hamstrings. It can be practiced using modifications similar to those in Viparita Karani, with a bolster, with a bolster and a folded blanket, or without any supports. And it's a nice option for someone who prefers less of an inversion.

BASIC "LEGS UP THE CHAIR" POSE

Basic "Legs up the Chair" Pose is the mini-variation of Viparita Karani. The only difference is that the lower legs are resting on a chair, and the upper legs are at an oblique angle to the torso rather than the legs being stretched straight up a wall.

How to Move into Basic "Legs up the Chair" Pose

1. Position a sturdy chair on the mat with the back of the chair facing you.
2. Have a bolster nearby.
3. Lie on your back, and rest the lower legs on the seat of the chair with the backs of the knees touching the lip of the seat.
4. Press the lower legs against the seat of the chair to lift the hips up, and then slide the bolster underneath the pelvis and lower back.

5. Allow the lower body to sink into gravity.
6. Breathe and relax.

How to Come out of Basic "Legs up the Chair" Pose

1. Lift the hips to remove any support underneath them.
2. Draw the knees in to the chest.
3. Roll to one side.
4. Pause.
5. Prepare for what's next.

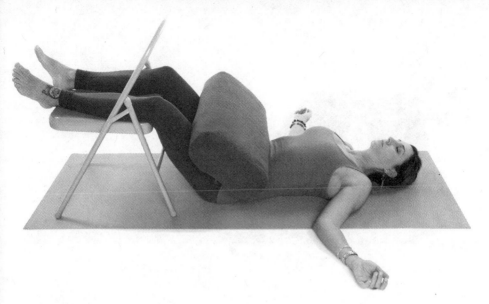

"LEGS UP THE CHAIR" POSE, VAR. 1

A little bit of weight on the top thighs helps to "ground" the pelvis and lower back in variation 1 of "Legs up the Chair" Pose. This is a nice option for someone who has an achy lower back. The added weight of a bolster helps to relax the lower back muscles. This is typically a valid option for everyone.

How to Move into "Legs up the Chair" Pose, Var. 1

1. Follow the basic pose instructions (page 81) with modified prop placement.
2. Breathe and relax.

How to Come out of "Legs up the Chair" Pose, Var. 1

Follow the basic pose instructions (page 82).

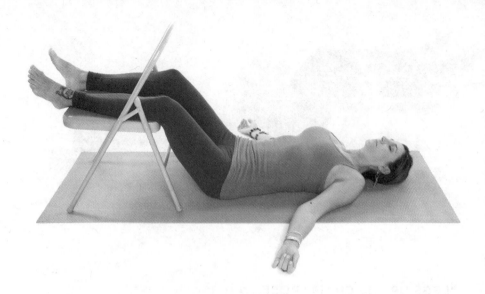

"LEGS UP THE CHAIR" POSE, VAR. 2

Variation 2 of "Legs up the Chair" Pose, which involves no support or weight for the pelvis or lower back, is a simple way to relieve lower body fatigue and melt away the daily stressors.

How to Move into "Legs up the Chair" Pose, Var. 2

1. Follow the basic pose instructions (page 81), omitting any use of a bolster.
2. Breathe and relax.

How to Come out of "Legs up the Chair" Pose, Var. 2

Follow steps 2 through 5 of the basic pose instructions (page 82).

CHAPTER 6

CALMING: FORWARD BENDS

....

Yapana forward bends are designed to cool the central nervous system and to deeply promote the "rest and digest" response.

The Yapana BEING forward-bend poses can create space in the hips, pelvis, and lower back. They may be very challenging for beginning students with a posterior-tilted pelvis or tight hamstrings, hip flexors, or lower back. Because they are designed to cool the central nervous system and to deeply promote "rest and digestion," strategic prop placement is crucial for maintaining SAS and physical comfort in the pose. Sometimes you may have to make the choice of giving up one thing to get something else. Ask yourself: what purpose does the forward bend serve? Your answer will determine the direction you pursue.

THREE IMPORTANT RULES TO FOLLOW WHEN PRACTICING FORWARD BENDS

1. **BE MINDFUL OF THE SPINE'S EXTENSION.** The practitioner must have two-thirds extension of the spine going into the pose before allowing flexion. That is, the lower back must lengthen, not flex and round, during the first two-thirds of the way into the pose. After that, the mid back can flex as much as needed; however, it is recommended that, to lengthen the back body, the chest and sternum move forward as much as they can comfortably.

2. **USE THE ARMS ONLY MINIMALLY IN THESE POSES.** Keep the arms out of the equation once settled in the pose. Do not use them to reach forward beyond the initial extension into the pose. There is no "achieving" in a BEING pose. Do not hold on to the feet to increase the stretch. If the arms don't reach the ground, use props to support them.

3. **BE MINDFUL OF THE ACTION IN THE LOWER LEGS.** The lower legs do not need to be firm to maintain alignment and SAS, but they should be held straight on their centerlines to prevent collapsing out to the sides.

4. **ALWAYS SUPPORT THE HEAD IN FORWARD BENDS.** The head should *always* be supported in forward bends. This is an important component to the level of relaxation in all BEING forward bends. Releasing the weight of the head into gravity in a downward position prevents the neck and upper back muscles from firing to hold up the head's weight in the forward-bend position. This is calming to the front of the brain.

General Contraindications for Forward Bends

- Hamstring injury — consult a qualified yoga therapist
- Sciatica — proceed with caution
- Sacroiliac joint dysfunction
- Pregnancy — avoid constricting the abdomen

General Benefits of Forward Bends

- Calm the brain
- Improve digestion
- Reduce fatigue
- Improve high blood pressure

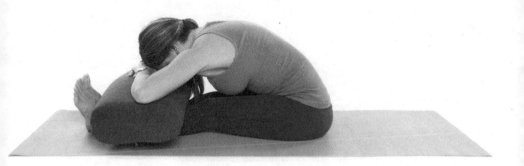

BASIC PASCHIMOTTANASANA
(SEATED FORWARD BEND POSE)

If your hip hinge is healthy, you don't need a lot of support to be comfortable and still in Basic Paschimottanasana.

How to Move into Basic Paschimottanasana

1. Sit upright and directly on the buttock bones with a bolster across the lower legs.
2. Lift the arms up alongside the head while keeping the lower ribs in and down.
3. Hinge forward at the hips while keeping the weight of your lower body sinking into the floor.
4. Hold on to the legs or feet while initially working the spine forward and down, keeping a flat back two-thirds of the way down before flexing.
5. Stretch both sides of the trunk evenly forward, and relax the forehead on the arms or on a bolster placed across the legs.
6. Breathe and relax.

How to Come out of Basic Paschimottanasana

1. Lift out of the pose either with a flat back or by rolling out vertebra by vertebra.
2. Pause.
3. Prepare for what's next.

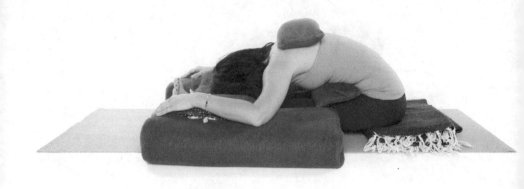

PASCHIMOTTANASANA, VAR. 1
(SEATED FORWARD BEND POSE, VAR. 1)

The strongest of the Paschimottanasana variations, variation 1 is great for someone with excellent flexibility who wishes to drop deep into the fold. Two sandbags are used: one placed across the shoulder blades for added release to the upper back and shoulders, and one placed across the top thighs to weigh down the legs and pelvis. To make sure the head is on the same plane as the chest, place a doubled-folded blanket underneath the head. Bolsters are placed on either side of the legs and are used as arm support. If you have the flexibility and stability for this variation, two words: *go inside.*

How to Move into Paschimottanasana, Var. 1

1. Follow the basic pose instructions (page 87) with modified prop placement.
2. Breathe and relax.

How to Come out of Paschimottanasana, Var. 1

Follow the basic pose instructions (page 87).

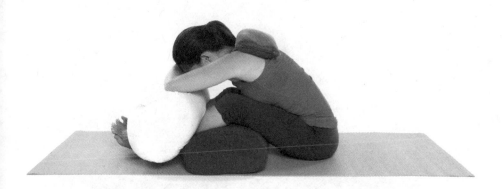

PASCHIMOTTANASANA, VAR. 2
(SEATED FORWARD BEND POSE, VAR. 2)

In variation 2 of Paschimottanasana, the use of a bolster underneath the knees and thighs supports tight hamstrings and offers a mild mid back stretch. This variation, however, makes sense only if you can sit forward on the buttock bones. This really is the key to bending from the hips (hip hinge) rather than the lower back. You must be able to sit upright with your weight toward the front of the buttock bones, indicating that the pelvis is in either a neutral or an anterior starting position. Another bolster is placed on top of the lower legs so that the arms and head can rest rather than reach.

How to Move into Paschimottanasana, Var. 2

1. Follow the basic pose instructions (page 87) with modified prop placement.
2. Breathe and relax.

How to Come out of Paschimottanasana, Var. 2

Follow the basic pose instructions (page 87).

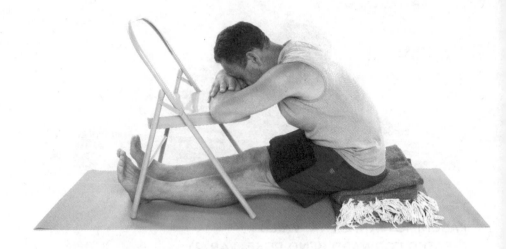

PASCHIMOTTANASANA, VAR. 3
(SEATED FORWARD BEND POSE, VAR. 3)

Using the seat of a chair in front of you for support while sitting on some height encourages the anterior pelvic tilt that's needed for moving into all forward bends. Greeting flexibility challenges rather than pushing against them in the BEING variations of classic poses such as variation 3 of Paschimottanasana is an act of kindness.

How to Move into Paschimottanasana, Var. 3

1. Follow the basic pose instructions (page 87) with modified prop placement.
2. Breathe and relax.

How to Come out of Paschimottanasana, Var. 3

Follow the basic pose instructions (page 87).

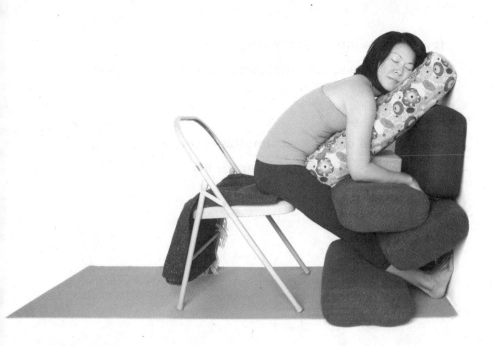

PASCHIMOTTANASANA, VAR. 4
(SEATED FORWARD BEND POSE, VAR. 4)

Let's say you are a student with a tight lower back and hamstrings. Perhaps you have a difficult time sitting upright without bending your knees or flexing at your lower back. Variation 4 of Paschimottanasana greatly elevates your pelvis, giving you the angle needed in order to be positioned on the front edge of the buttock bones and find some length in the lower back. In addition to the use of a chair for the added height, a bolster is placed on the floor a few inches away from the wall. The soles of the feet are positioned against the wall and the calves against the bolster. Once you are in the forward bend, the support offers a generous stretch to the calves. Stack up additional bolsters on top of the legs so that they meet you and you don't lose the length in the lower back.

If you determine that getting a safe stretch in the hamstrings is needed more than the deep relaxation benefits of having the head lower, this is a safe and logical variation.

How to Move into Paschimottanasana, Var. 4

1. Follow the basic pose instructions (page 87) with modified prop placement.
2. Breathe and relax.

How to Come out of Paschimottanasana, Var. 4

Follow the basic pose instructions (page 87).

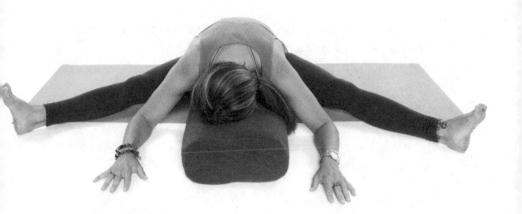

BASIC UPAVISTA KONASANA
(SEATED WIDE-ANGLE POSE)

Do you wonder why you are challenged in a seated forward bend when the legs are together but less so when they are apart? Easy, it's your hamstrings. The hamstrings are made up of two muscles (semitendinosus and semimembranosus) that run medially, or on the inner side of the thighbone, and one muscle (biceps femoris) that runs laterally, or on the outer side of the thighbone. When the legs are closer together, the lateral hamstrings receive the greatest stretch. When the legs are farther apart, the medial hamstrings receive the greatest stretch.

Most people have imbalances in which the medial muscles are looser than the lateral muscles, or vice versa. Therefore, you may find that your forward bend with legs close together is more challenging than when you separate your legs. Also, separating your legs may give you a little more room in your hips to move into a better neutral starting pelvic position. Each of these variations meets several levels of flexibility.

How to Move into Basic Upavista Konasana

1. Sit down with the legs stretched out to the sides close to 90° apart.
2. Place the short end of a bolster against the pelvis and belly.
3. Stretch the arms overhead and lengthen the waist, grow long, and sit up taller.

4. Stretch forward to rest the torso and head on top of the bolster, turning the head in one direction or the other.
5. Keep your hips releasing into the floor.
6. Breathe and relax.

How to Come out of Basic Upavista Konasana

1. Lift out of the pose either with a flat back or by rolling out vertebra by vertebra.
2. Pause.
3. Prepare for what's next.

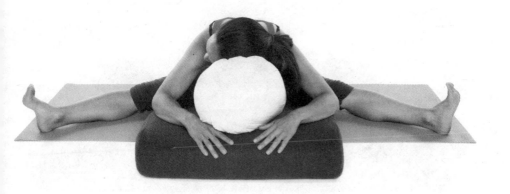

UPAVISTA KONASANA, VAR. 1
(SEATED WIDE-ANGLE POSE, VAR. 1)

Variation 1 of Upavista Konasana is a simple modification of the basic pose using two bolsters stacked in a T formation with the arms loosely draped over the bottom bolster. Bring the top bolster all the way up against the pelvis and belly for total support. It's that easy.

How to Move into Upavista Konasana, Var. 1

1. Follow the basic pose instructions (page 93) with modified prop placement.
2. Breathe and relax.

How to Come out of Upavista Konasana, Var. 1

Follow the basic pose instructions (page 94).

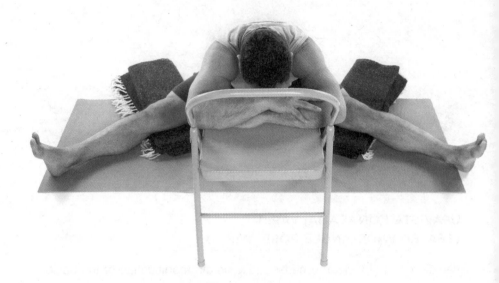

UPAVISTA KONASANA, VAR. 2
(SEATED WIDE-ANGLE POSE, VAR. 2)

If you need considerable support underneath your pelvis to sit upright easily, it may put quite a bit of space between the backs of the legs and the floor. In variation 2 of Upavista Konasana, the legs are supported to prevent them from hovering and to provide feedback underneath them so they can relax. If you are better at hinging forward with a lot of support underneath your hips, you are probably a candidate who also does better with the height of a chair seat for upper body and arm support. You'll be giving up the cushioned support of a bolster being right up against you, but you will be maintaining the important hip hinge skill for safe alignment.

How to Move into Upavista Konasana, Var. 2

1. Follow the basic pose instructions (page 93) with modified prop placement.
2. Breathe and relax.

How to Come out of Upavista Konasana, Var. 2

Follow the basic pose instructions (page 94).

CHAPTER 7

OTHER POSE OPTIONS

....

A BEING practice can help us to honor and value the breath rather than the depth of stretch.

The following poses consist of those that are practiced seated, side lying, supine (on your back), or prone (on your belly). The seated and side-lying poses stretch the sides of the body. The supine and prone poses are considered "hip openers," as they stretch the legs and hips, with the exception of one shoulder stretch on your back.

SEATED POSES

General Contraindications

- Knee injury
- Hamstring injury
- Groin injury

General Benefits

- Stimulate abdominal organs
- Improve digestion

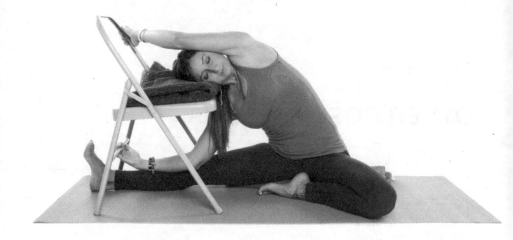

BASIC PARIVRTTA JANU SIRSASANA
(REVOLVED HEAD TO KNEE POSE)

Basic Parivrtta Janu Sirsasana is a challenging pose for many, but practicing it with support makes it accessible for most. The only way to stretch the front, back, and side of the waist at the same time is to practice a side bend, and this always involves stretching an arm overhead and flexing at the waist. The quadratus lumborum, an important postural muscle that rests deep in the back of the waist, receives a tremendous stretch here. With the exception of a few standing and seated poses and Balasana (Child Pose) variations, no other pose targets the back of the waist like a side bend. If you sit for prolonged periods of time, this muscle can get very short and tight.

The challenge (and magic) of this pose is balancing the side stretch and gentle rotation of the chest without lifting the pelvis off the floor. Consider placing a blanket underneath the seat to help maintain a neutral pelvic position. When the head reaches the chair, it should be on the same general plane as the chest rather than falling off the top of the spine or struggling to meet the height of the chair seat. If the seat of the chair is too low for the head to meet it, you can build up its height with more blankets, but you risk losing the length in the waist. If that happens, raise the chair on blocks so that you are working with the chair at an appropriate height for the height of your body.

There may be a tendency to "work" this pose. Refrain from doing so. Once you find the right support, the pose will encourage your "heart space" to shine and any heaviness to melt away.

How to Move into Basic Parivrtta Janu Sirsasana

1. At one end of the mat, position a sturdy chair with a folded blanket on its seat.
2. Stretch the right leg through the bottom frame of the chair, and bring the left foot in toward the pelvis, as in Baddha Konasana (Bound Angle Pose), and consider placing a meditation pad underneath the left buttock if it is hovering.
3. Hold on to the bottom rung of the chair with the right hand.
4. Lengthen the waist before stretching the left arm overhead to reach for the farther side of the chair's reinforcement bar.
5. Rest the head on the blanket, and turn the chest toward the sky.
6. Relax and breathe.

How to Come out of Basic Parivrtta Janu Sirsasana

1. Release both hands to stretch up and into an upright position.
2. Pause.
3. Prepare for the opposite side.

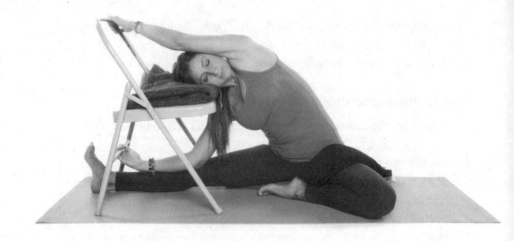

PARIVRTTA JANU SIRSASANA, VAR. 1
(REVOLVED HEAD TO KNEE POSE, VAR. 1)

If stretching the top arm proves difficult in Basic Parivṛtta Janu Sirsasana, reduce the reach in variation 1 by holding on to any part of the
chair's reinforcement bar. "Grounding" the bent leg with weight is always
an option and actually helps to stretch the side body even more and
assists the top arm in its role to stretch and reach.

How to Move into Parivrtta Janu Sirsasana, Var. 1

1. Follow the basic pose instructions (page 99) with modified prop
   placement.
2. Breathe and relax.

How to Come out of Parivrtta Janu Sirsasana, Var. 1

Follow the basic pose instructions (page 99).

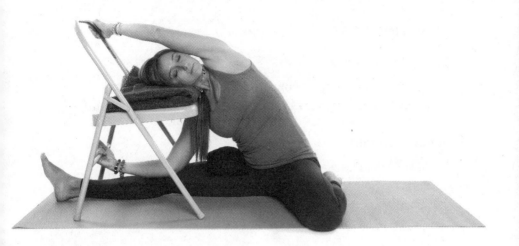

PARIVRTTA JANU SIRSASANA, VAR. 2
(REVOLVED HEAD TO KNEE POSE, VAR. 2)

If the hamstrings of the straight leg need a little more flexibility support in Parivrtta Janu Sirsasana, placing a 10-pound sandbag across the upper thigh is an excellent option in variation 2. The more flexibility coming from the straight leg, the better access to a safe hip hinge in this pose. Also in this variation, you can adjust the bent leg into another position, such as Virasana (Hero Pose), as shown above. Ask yourself what you need and why.

How to Move into Parivrtta Janu Sirsasana, Var. 2

Follow the basic pose instructions (page 99) but with the modified weight placement and perhaps the modified position of the bent leg.

How to Come out of Parivrtta Janu Sirsasana, Var. 2

Follow the basic pose instructions (page 99).

SIDE-LYING POSES

General Contraindications

- Serious back injury — consult a qualified yoga therapist
- Serious shoulder injury — modify placement of bottom arm

General Benefits

- Relieve mild backaches
- Improve rib cage mobility

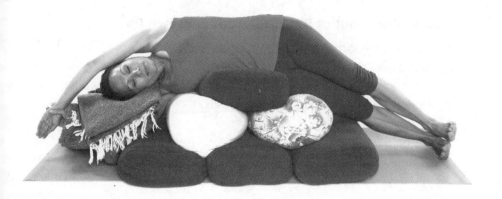

BASIC SIDE-LYING STRETCH POSE

The basic side-lying stretch pose, along with its variations, is a small alteration of Parivrtta Janu Sirsasana (Revolved Head to Knee Pose) without the work in the legs. The BEING versions of this pose are excellent opportunities to passively attend to muscle tightness on all sides of the waist and rib cage. Let the stretch percolate over time. As in many other poses, the head should be supported on the same plane as the chest so that it stays in alignment with the spine.

How to Move into Basic Side-Lying Stretch Pose

1. Prepare the bolster support as in Basic Viparita Dandasana (Basic Inverted Two-Legged Staff Pose) (page 55).
2. Lean the right side onto the support, and place a folded blanket between the bottom arm and the head.
3. Stretch the right arm, so that the sides of the waist are well stretched.
4. Stretch the left arm overhead, using the right hand to take hold of the left wrist.
5. Straighten the legs, and rest the head on the blanket.
6. Breathe and relax.

How to Come out of Basic Side-Lying Stretch Pose

1. Release the top arm, and rest it on the top hip.
2. Bend the knees.
3. Lean the chest toward the support, and use the hands to push up and sit back in a comfortable position.
4. Pause.
5. Prepare for the opposite side.

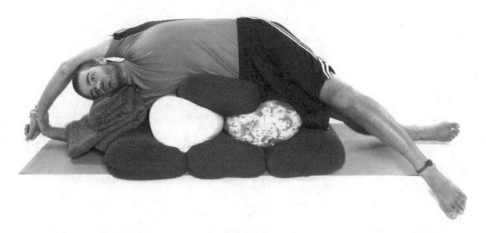

SIDE-LYING STRETCH POSE, VAR. 1

In variation 1 of Side-Lying Stretch Pose, simply changing the legs into a "scissor"-legged position, where the top leg stretches forward of the bottom leg, can provide a stretch to the iliotibial band (IT band), a large tendon that runs along the outer legs. Part of the IT band's job is to stabilize the outer knee joint, so a tight IT band can result in knee pain. This tendon is easily overused in running, walking, and cycling, so people who engage in these activities may benefit from this variation.

How to Move into Side-Lying Stretch Pose, Var. 1

1. Follow the basic pose instructions (page 103) with modified positioning of the legs.
2. Breathe and relax.

How to Come out of Side-Lying Stretch Pose, Var. 1

Follow the basic pose instructions (page 104).

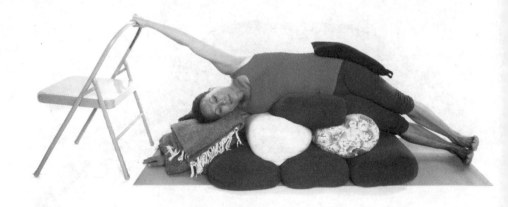

SIDE-LYING STRETCH POSE, VAR. 2

Less is more. In Basic Side-Lying Stretch Pose and its variation 1, does the top arm have a difficult time reaching overhead without the shoulders or back becoming rounded? Shoulders can be inflexible for myriad reasons, but because the Side-Lying Stretch Pose is also a side-bending pose, the latissimi dorsi (lateral back muscles) may be the culprit in this case. If these muscles are tight, they limit the range of motion in the shoulders. In variation 2, modify the height of the support for the top arm as much as necessary, such as using a chair back for that arm to rest on, or even keep the top arm out of the stretch altogether. Not engaging the top arm, however, will lessen the side stretch. Choose wisely.

How to Move into Side-Lying Stretch Pose, Var. 2

1. Follow the basic pose instructions (page 103) with modified prop placement or top arm involvement.
2. Breathe and relax.

How to Come out of Side-Lying Stretch Pose, Var. 2

Follow the basic pose instructions (page 104).

SUPINE STANDING POSES

Supine variations of standing poses offer a unique opportunity to stretch areas that may be bypassed when the poses are performed with the body upright. They provide a wonderful way to understand personal alignment without being in a weight-bearing position.

General Contraindications

- SI joint dysfunction — consult a qualified yoga therapist
- Hamstring injury
- Groin injury

General Benefits

- Improve digestion
- Help to alleviate general back pain

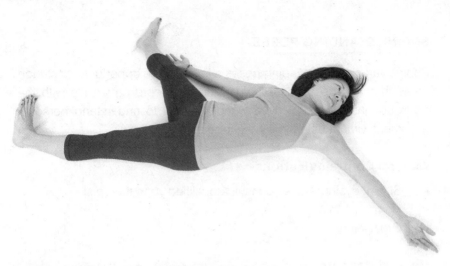

BASIC SUPTA UTTHITA TRIKONASANA (RECLINING EXTENDED TRIANGLE POSE)

Extended Triangle on the floor — prepare for a delicious stretch! The wall and the floor provide excellent feedback for finding a neutral pelvis. If you get confused, just imagine that your feet are standing on the floor and you are in the classic upright position.

How to Move into Basic Supta Utthita Trikonasana

1. Lie down on the floor near a wall, and position the feet approximately 3½ to 4½ feet apart where the floor and wall meet, rotating the right foot out 90° and turning the left foot in about 15°.
2. Gently push your legs away from your center and stretch your arms out into a T position.
3. Lengthen your waist, hinge at the right hip, and slide your torso and right arm to the right.
4. When you cannot flex any farther, lower your right hand to the front leg and reach your left arm out with the palm facing upward.
5. Either turn the head to look over the left arm or keep it in a neutral position.
6. Breathe and relax.

How to Come out of Basic Supta Utthita Trikonasana

1. Bend the left knee, and place the foot on the floor.
2. Draw the left arm in to the chest.
3. Roll to the right side.
4. Pause.
5. Prepare for the opposite side.

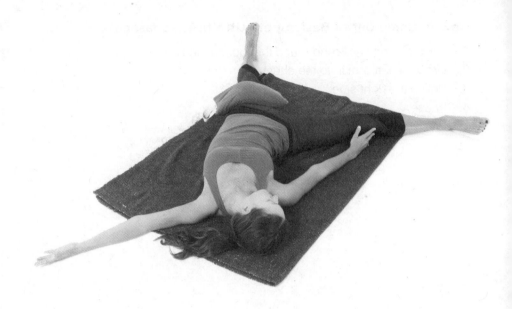

SUPTA UTTHITA TRIKONASANA, VAR. 1
(RECLINING EXTENDED TRIANGLE POSE, VAR. 1)

When Utthita Trikonasana is practiced upright, if the back rounds, it may be a sign of either poor muscle flexibility or weakness. Using a 10-pound sandbag on top of the back thigh addresses the flexibility issue by slowly increasing the stretch of that leg. The added weight helps to keep the mid buttock on the ground, which promotes an even stretch across the front of the hips.

How to Move into Supta Utthita Trikonasana, Var. 1

1. Follow the basic pose instructions (page 108) with modified prop placement.
2. Breathe and relax.

How to Come out of Supta Utthita Trikonasana, Var. 1

Follow the basic pose instructions (page 109).

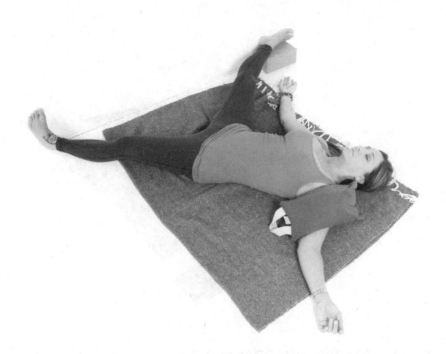

SUPTA UTTHITA TRIKONASANA, VAR. 2
(RECLINING EXTENDED TRIANGLE POSE, VAR. 2)

In the pose, both shoulders should remain on the floor so that the stretch across the front of the chest and the shoulders themselves is equal. In variation 2, a 10-pound sandbag is placed across the left shoulder, which, because of the pose's trajectory, is the one that receives the greatest stretch. Also, the front foot is shown elevated. The elevation keeps weight equally distributed on both mid buttocks and keeps the stretch from loading in the knee.

How to Move into Supta Utthita Trikonasana, Var. 2

1. Follow the basic pose instructions (page 108) with modified prop placement.
2. Breathe and relax.

How to Come out of Supta Utthita Trikonasana, Var. 2

Follow the basic pose instructions (page 109).

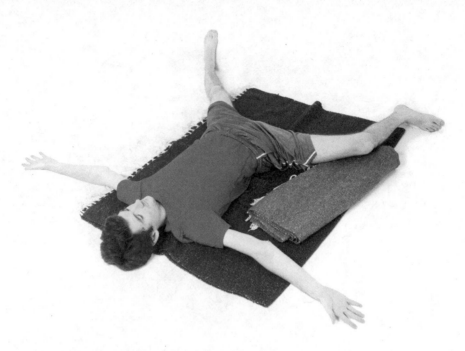

BASIC SUPTA VIRABHADRASANA 2
(RECLINING WARRIOR 2 POSE)

Similar to Supta Utthita Trikonasana (Reclining Extended Triangle Pose), Supta Virabhadrasana 2 stretches the front of the pelvis, hips, and legs, and both mid buttocks should remain on the floor. If the knee of the bent leg is hovering more than an inch or two off the floor, place support underneath it so that the muscles can receive feedback to relax.

How to Move into Basic Supta Virabhadrasana 2

1. Lie down on the floor near a wall, and position the feet approximately 3½ to 4½ feet apart where the floor and wall meet, rotating the right foot out 90° and turning the left foot in about 15°.
2. Bend the right leg into a 90° angle, and slide closer to the wall if necessary to find proper alignment.
3. Stretch the arms into a T position with the palms turned upward.
4. Drop the bottom of the front ribs.
5. Either turn the head to look over the right arm or keep it in a neutral position.
6. Breathe and relax.

How to Come out of Basic Supta Virabhadrasana 2

1. Bend the left knee, and place that foot on the floor.
2. Draw the left arm in to the chest.
3. Roll to the right side.
4. Pause.
5. Prepare for the opposite side.

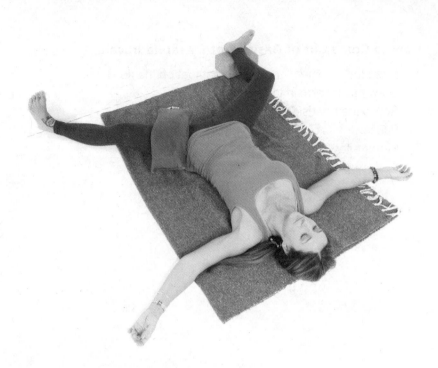

SUPTA VIRABHADRASANA 2, VAR. 1
(RECLINING WARRIOR 2 POSE, VAR. 1)

Typically, in Supta Virabhadrasana 2 if the knee of the bent leg is higher than the hip line, the foot should be elevated with a block. Otherwise, the weight of gravity will settle in the front hip and eventually load unequally in the lower back. Also in variation 1 of this pose, a 10-pound sandbag is placed on the back leg to help weight it.

How to Move into Supta Virabhadrasana 2, Var. 1

1. Follow the basic pose instructions (page 112) with modified prop placement.
2. Breathe and relax.

How to Come out of Supta Virabhadrasana 2, Var. 1

Follow the basic pose instructions (page 113).

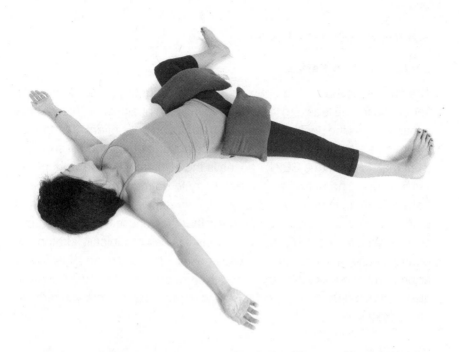

SUPTA VIRABHADRASANA 2, VAR. 2
(RECLINING WARRIOR 2 POSE, VAR. 2)

For the ultimate passive hip opener, variation 2 of Supta Virabhadrasana 2, try a sandbag on each thigh. The only candidates for variation 2 of this pose are those who can easily keep the knee of the bent leg on the same plane as the hip. Basically, the front knee should not be hovering aboveground. Once this alignment is achieved, the sandbags provide welcome props that release the hips for a deep opening.

How to Move into Supta Virabhadrasana 2, Var. 2

1. Follow the basic pose instructions (page 112) with modified prop placement.
2. Breathe and relax.

How to Come out of Supta Virabhadrasana 2, Var. 2

Follow the basic pose instructions (page 113).

SUPINE POSES FOR LEGS

Leg Stretching Series

The supine poses for legs can be practiced together as a therapeutic sequence for the legs and lower back. Since the health of the hamstrings in part informs the health of the lower back, each pose offers an opportunity to safely stretch the hamstrings. Besides the obvious prop support, what makes them true BEING poses is the elimination of the work of the arms. There is no pulling on the belt to try to do more. Simply adjust the belt's tension to increase or decrease the stretch. Sometimes we have to actively choose to do less on our mat rather than chase the greatest sensations. With the right support, your muscles can organically stretch out during meaningful time spent in these poses. This may bring a newfound approach to your practice that not only supports the life of the pose but also fosters a deeper relationship with your practice and how you receive and perceive it.

General Contraindications

- Hamstring injury
- Groin injury

General Benefits

- Improve digestion
- Relieve backaches
- Ease menstrual cramps

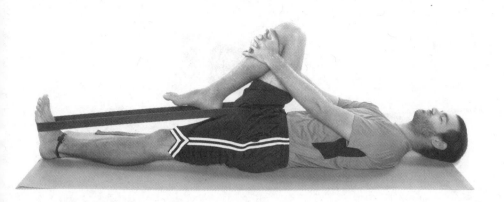

BASIC ARDHA APANASANA
(HALF KNEE TO CHEST POSE)

Basic Ardha Apanasana can provide traction to the lower back through the dynamic tension created by looping a belt around the foot of the straight leg and the thigh of the bent leg.

How to Move into Basic Ardha Apanasana

1. Adjust the loop of a fastened yoga belt so that it's the length of the entire leg, and place it nearby.
2. Lie down on your back, and bend the right leg.
3. Place the belt around the sole of the left foot and the top thigh of the right leg (near the hip crease).
4. Catch the upper shin of the right leg with the hands, and draw the leg in toward the chest. Be sure to adjust the belt as necessary to maintain a level of tension between the two legs without hindering the flexion of the right hip and knee.
5. Stretch the tailbone toward the left foot to lengthen the lower back.
6. Breathe and relax.

How to Come out of Basic Ardha Apanasana

1. Release the bent leg, and set that foot on the ground.
2. Bend the opposite leg.
3. Pause.
4. Prepare for the opposite side.

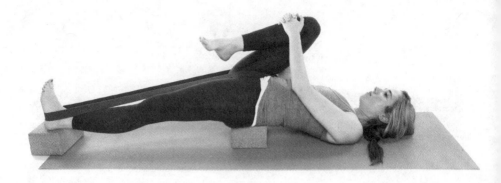

ARDHA APANASANA, VAR. 1
(HALF KNEE TO CHEST POSE, VAR. 1)

Variation 1 of Ardha Apanasana is an awesome way to target the hip flexors (muscles on the front side of the hip joint). Elevating the pelvis with a block changes the plane between the pelvis and the shoulders, offering a stretch to the quadriceps and hip flexors. This variation shows a block underneath the foot of the straight leg just in case the elevated pelvis creates a shortening in the lower back.

How to Move into Ardha Apanasana, Var. 1

1. Follow the basic pose instructions (page 117) with modified prop placement.
2. Breathe and relax.

How to Come out of Ardha Apanasana, Var. 1

1. Release the bent leg, and set that foot on the floor.
2. Bend the opposite leg.
3. Push the feet against the floor to lift the pelvis, and slide the block out from underneath it.
4. Pause.
5. Prepare for the opposite side.

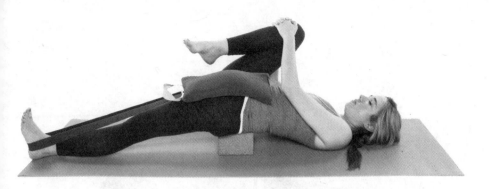

ARDHA APANASANA, VAR. 2
(HALF KNEE TO CHEST POSE, VAR. 2)

Variation 2 of Ardha Apanasana takes the pose up a notch by eliminating the block underneath the foot of the straight leg and placing a 10-pound sandbag on that top thigh. The combination of lowering the foot so that the pelvis is the highest point in the pose and adding the weight offers the deepest stretch to the flexors of all three Ardha Apanasana poses.

How to Move into Ardha Apanasana, Var. 2

1. Follow the basic pose instructions (page 117) with modified prop placement.
2. Breathe and relax.

How to Come out of Ardha Apanasana, Var. 2

Follow the basic pose instructions for variation 1 (page 118).

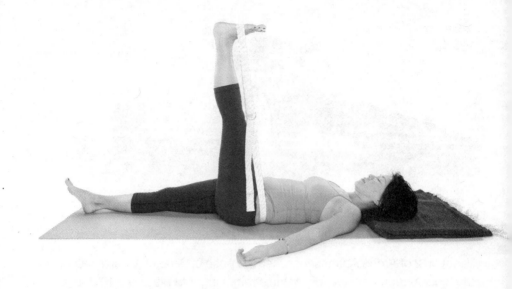

BASIC SUPTA PADANGUSTHASANA 1
(RECLINING BIG TOE 1 POSE)

Like Ardha Apanasana (Half Knee to Chest Pose), the BEING pose Supta Padangusthasana creates traction and balances both sides of the lower back. The floor is the perfect feedback for how the hamstrings play a role in the position of the pelvis. When you stretch the leg up to the ceiling, notice how the pelvis tilts either forward or backward depending on how close you bring the leg to the torso. Keep the leg straight while maintaining a neutral pelvic position. The belt is placed around the lower back to stabilize the stretch by drawing the leg into the pelvis.

How to Move into Basic Supta Padangusthasana 1

1. Adjust the loop of a fastened yoga belt so that it's the length of the entire leg, and place it nearby.
2. Lie supine on the floor with the knees bent.
3. Place the belt around the lower back and the sole of the left foot, and then extend that leg to the ceiling.
4. Stretch the right leg downward from the torso.
5. Relax the arms alongside the body with the palms turned upward.
6. Breathe and relax.

How to Come out of Basic Supta Padangusthasana 1

1. Bend the raised leg, hug that knee in to the chest a few moments, and then place that foot on the floor.
2. Bend the bottom leg, and place that foot on the floor.
3. Pause.
4. Prepare for the opposite side.

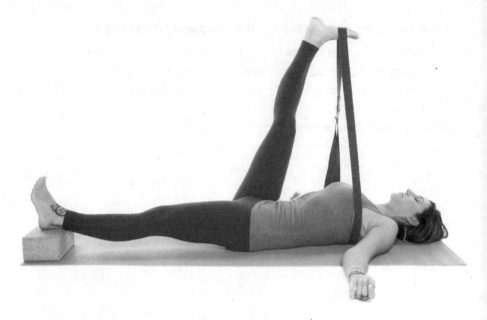

SUPTA PADANGUSTHASANA 1, VAR. 1
(RECLINING BIG TOE 1 POSE, VAR. 1)

If the raised leg in Supta Padangusthasana can stretch beyond a 90° position, then slide the belt up to the mid or upper back. The angle will provide a stronger pull on the leg, but if the leg naturally stretches beyond the 90° position, then the hamstrings can handle it. You always have the option to place a block underneath the foot of the lower leg to avoid any pull on the lower back.

How to Move into Supta Padangusthasana 1, Var. 1

1. Follow the basic pose instructions (page 120) with modified prop placement.
2. Breathe and relax.

How to Come out of Supta Padangusthasana 1, Var. 1

Follow the basic pose instructions (page 121).

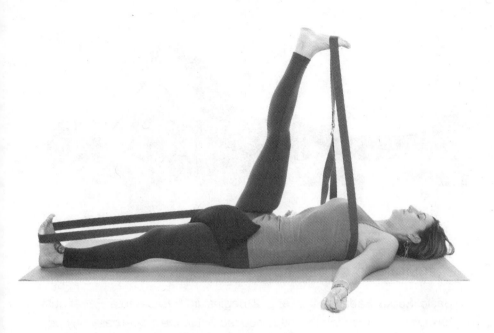

SUPTA PADANGUSTHASANA 1, VAR. 2
(RECLINING BIG TOE 1 POSE, VAR. 2)

Variation 2 of Supta Padangusthasana is very supportive to hamstring and hip flexor flexibility, and of all the variations, it provides the greatest amount of traction to the lower back. In addition to the belt around the torso and the foot of the raised leg, a belt around the foot of the lower leg and the thigh of the raised leg gives the perfect feedback to foster lower back relief from a compressed spine.

How to Move into Supta Padangusthasana 1, Var. 2

1. Follow the basic pose instructions (page 120) with modified prop placement.
2. Breathe and relax.

How to Come out of Supta Padangusthasana 1, Var. 2

Follow the basic pose instructions (page 121).

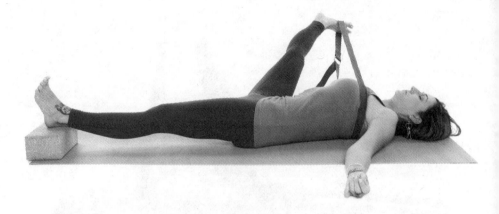

BASIC SUPTA PADANGUSTHASANA 2
(RECLINING BIG TOE 2 POSE)

Basic Supta Padangusthasana 2 begins in Basic Supta Padangusthasana 1 and then rotates the raised leg out to the side. There may be a
tendency to throw the leg out as if it were disconnected from the body's
center. Instead, while you are moving the leg out, consider ways in which
your movement integrates the stretch into your center rather than pulling
away from it.

If the BEING poses are adequately supported, you can spend more than
just five or ten breaths in them. They are not meant to take you to your
physical edge from the get-go. I'm not saying you aren't going to feel
sensations or that you shouldn't. I'm saying that if you practice moving
in and out of this and other BEING poses with an interest in generating
sukha (happy/good space), you will be in balance with what the Yapana
style of practice is teaching.

You can use support for the raised leg to rest against or not. The belt is
positioned as it was in Supta Padangusthasana 1, Var. 1 (page 122). And
a block is underneath the foot of the leg that's on the floor, to manage the
degree of stretch in the lower back.

How to Move into Basic Supta Padangusthasana 2

1. Place a double-folded blanket or bolster to the right of the mat,
    and a block on the left side of the foot end of the mat.

2. Take Basic Supta Padangusthasana 1 (page 120), with a block underneath the left foot to keep the stretch in the lower back to a minimum.
3. Turn the right thighbone out (in an external rotation), and simultaneously stretch that leg to the right to rest it on the blanket or bolster support.

How to Come out of Basic Supta Padangusthasana 2

1. Stretch the leg back into Basic Supta Padangusthasana 1.
2. Bend the raised leg, hug that knee in to the chest a few moments, and then place that foot on the floor.
3. Bend the bottom leg, and place that foot on the floor.
4. Pause.
5. Prepare for the opposite side.

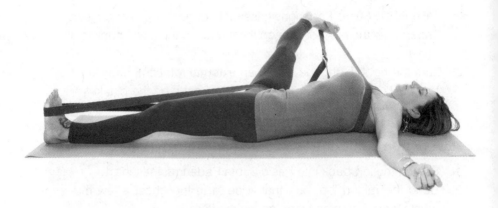

SUPTA PADANGUSTHASANA 2, VAR. 1
(RECLINING BIG TOE 2 POSE, VAR. 1)

The variation of Supta Padangusthasana 2 is set up just like Supta Padangusthasana 1, Var. 2 (Reclining Big Toe 1 Pose, Var. 2). It provides a lot of feedback and support. The lower belt provides excellent feedback for maintaining an external rotation of the leg and a neutral pelvis, while the upper belt supports the stretch of the leg as it is being drawn in to the center.

How to Move into Supta Padangusthasana 2, Var. 1

1. Follow the basic pose instructions (page 124) with modified prop placement.
2. Breathe and relax.

How to Come out of Supta Padangusthasana 2, Var. 1

Follow the basic pose instructions (page 125).

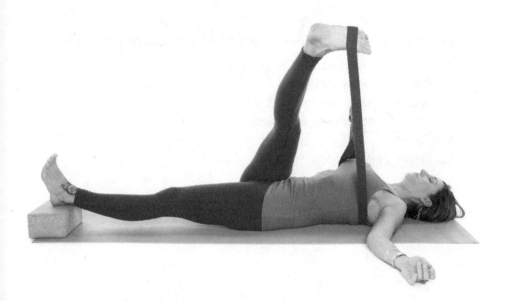

BASIC SUPTA PARIVRTTA PADANGUSTHASANA (RECLINING REVOLVED BIG TOE POSE)

This Supta Padangusthasana sequence began by stretching the front of the legs, followed by the back and inner legs, and now finishes with the outer legs. These poses may be practiced individually or in the series. Basic Supta Parivrtta Padangusthasana offers an opportunity to stretch the largest skeletal muscle in the body, the gluteus maximus (buttock). How close you can get the stretched leg to the floor is not important. The value of this pose is in keeping both sides of the lower back aligned and remaining in contact with the floor without being too rigid as your body responds to the movement of the breath and the changes in the stretch. The belt can be positioned at either the lower back or the mid back. If you feel challenged by hamstring stretches, position the belt at the lower back. If you can easily straighten your leg perpendicular to the mat, position the belt at the mid back.

How to Move into Basic Supta Parivrtta Padangusthasana

1. Start in Basic Supta Padangusthasana 1 (page 120) with the belt positioned across your lower or mid back.
2. Turn the right thighbone out (in an external rotation), and simultaneously stretch it across the torso to the left.

How to Come out of Basic Supta Parivrtta Padangusthasana

1. Stretch the leg back into Basic Supta Padangusthasana 1.
2. Bend the top leg, hug that knee in to the chest a few moments, and then place that foot on the floor.
3. Bend the bottom leg, and place that foot on the floor.
4. Pause.
5. Prepare for the opposite side.

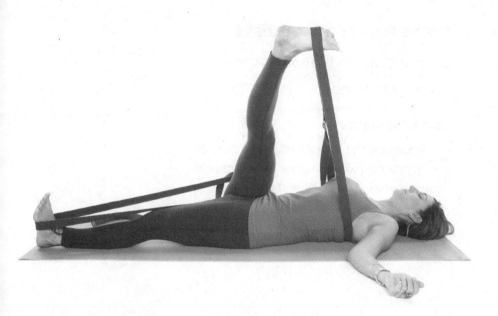

SUPTA PARIVRTTA PADANGUSTHASANA, VAR. 1
(RECLINING REVOLVED BIG TOE POSE, VAR. 1)

Do you see the pattern among the Supta Padangusthasana poses? Each variation within this series offers the exact setup that provides necessary feedback and support to stretch the legs, stabilize the pelvis, and keep safe alignment.

How to Move into Supta Parivrtta Padangusthasana, Var. 1

1. Follow the basic pose instructions (page 127) but with the addition of a second belt, around the bottom leg, as in Supta Padangusthasana 1, Var. 2 (page 123).
2. Breathe and relax.

How to Come out of Supta Parivrtta Padangusthasana, Var. 1

Follow the basic pose instructions (page 128).

SUPINE POSE FOR SHOULDERS

General Contraindication

- Shoulder injury

General Benefits

- Improves shoulder mobility and flexibility
- Improves mid and upper back mobility
- Relieves upper back and neck tension

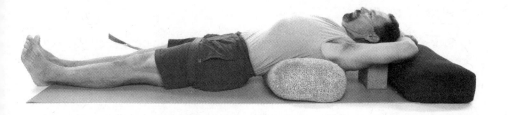

RECLINING SHOULDER STRETCH

Reclining Shoulder Stretch is a superb way to open the mid back and stretch the shoulders. A bolster supports the shoulder blades, another bolster supports the weight of the folded arms, and a block supports the head. Awesome!

How to Move into Reclining Shoulder Stretch

1. Position two bolsters across your mat — one bolster at the top end and the other nearer the center of the mat with approximately 8 inches of space between the two. Position the block on edge in between.
2. Stretch your legs out, and fasten a yoga belt firmly around the top thighs.
3. Sit approximately 6 inches in front of the bottom bolster.
4. Place the hands on the floor on either side of your hips, and while lifting the chest, lie back until the shoulder blades touch the top edge of the bottom bolster and the head rests on the block.
5. Stretch your arms overhead, and then bend the arms and cradle an elbow in each hand. Reverse your elbow hold halfway through.
6. Breathe and relax.

How to Come out of Reclining Shoulder Stretch

1. Release the arms from overhead.
2. Bend the knees, and place the feet on the floor.
3. Draw the left arm in to your chest.
4. Push off with the feet, and roll to the right.
5. Pause.
6. Prepare for what's next.

PRONE POSES

Prone poses are another example of how props can be placed strategically to provide ample support for the most comfort. Positioning the body facedown is required in all prone poses, unlike most other poses, and may bring attention to stiffness and tension of which you are unaware. Just remember to breathe into what is happening while in the pose, and be ever mindful of SAS to prevent overstretching or misalignment.

General Contraindications

- Ankle injury
- Knee injury
- Groin injury
- SI joint dysfunction

General Benefits

- Increase blood flow to pelvic organs
- Relieve lower back pain
- Improve hip flexion flexibility

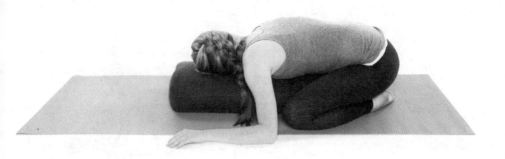

BASIC BALASANA (CHILD POSE)

Generally, Basic Balasana is loved by all, with the exception of those whose hips or knees or both cannot or should not hyperflex. It is the perfect pose to practice after a twist, as it settles the back into a neutral position, which is important after rotating the spine. It provides welcome relief for those with a tight lower back. One rule should be followed for this pose: the shoulders and hips are to be kept on the same plane — neither should be above or below the other. This ensures that the pose achieves a balance of flexibility between hip flexion and the lower back.

How to Move into Basic Balasana

1. Start in a table position on hands and knees, resting on the tops of the feet.
2. Position the legs widely enough for them to rest outside your side ribs, and slide a bolster between the legs.
3. Bend at the hips to bring the pelvis down to the heel bones while resting the torso on the bolster.
4. Turn the head to the right, so that the right nostril is on top.
5. Rest the arms in a goalpost position.

How to Come out of Basic Balasana

1. Keep the chin in a neutral position relative to a neutral skull.
2. Turn the head to rest the forehead on the bolster.
3. Place the hands on the floor underneath the shoulders, and straighten the arms to lift the torso away from the bolster.
4. Sit back on the heels or in any comfortable position.
5. Pause.
6. Prepare for what's next.

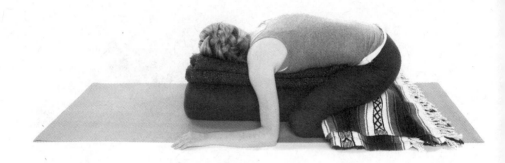

BALASANA, VAR. 1 (CHILD POSE, VAR. 1)

Variation 1 of Balasana is how you bring the pose to those who don't have the shoulders and hips on the same plane. Build the support up until this is achieved. If building up the torso support means that the hips still hover over the heels, consider placing a blanket near the tops of the thighs at the hip crease. An added blanket is also a good option for someone who requires less flexion in the knees. When using support for this purpose, place the long folded edge of the blanket all the way into the knee crease. And if the elbows hover and are no longer on the same plane as the hands, then fill that space with support, too.

How to Move into Balasana, Var. 1

1. Follow the basic pose instructions (page 133) with modified prop placement.
2. Breathe and relax.

How to Come out of Balasana, Var. 1

Follow the basic pose instructions (page 133).

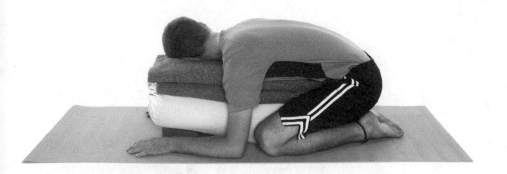

BALASANA, VAR. 2 (CHILD POSE, VAR. 2)

Another way to bring Balasana to the student is with variation 2, in which the top end of the support is elevated, creating a slight angle, as shown in the photograph above. I've added a few more double-folded blankets to fill the space between the body and the support. This is a good option if the hips are releasing but the torso still drops below the hip line.

How to Move into Balasana, Var. 2

1. Follow the basic pose instructions (page 133) with modified prop placement.
2. Breathe and relax.

How to Come out of Balasana, Var. 2

Follow the basic pose instructions (page 133).

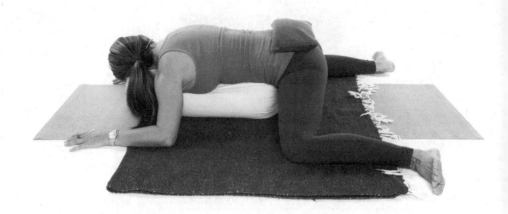

BASIC BHEKASANA (FROG POSE)

You either love to love Basic Bhekasana or love to avoid it. This pose offers a generous stretch to the adductors (inner thigh muscles), which are also considered balancing agents for our legs. We need them strong and flexible in order to walk and balance without falling over. As in Balasana (Child Pose), position the support to keep the shoulders and hips on the same plane when possible. Never overstretch. If the weight ends up loading a collapsed lower back or a dipped chest, keep exploring a better setup. Finding the right support may take some time, but it is well worth the effort and patience.

How to Move into Basic Bhekasana

1. Cover a yoga mat with a blanket to pad the knees, and place a bolster on the mat in a parallel orientation.
2. Start in a table position on hands and knees over the bolster.
3. Separate the legs wide apart, and rest the shins on the floor, parallel to the edges of the mat.
4. Rest the torso on the bolster, allowing the pelvis to hang off it, and place the arms in a goalpost position.
5. Turn the head to the right, so that the right nostril is on top.
6. Breathe and relax.

How to Come out of Basic Bhekasana

1. Rotate the ankles so that the toes turn under and point toward the tailbone.
2. Push the hands against the floor to pull your body forward, and straighten the legs.
3. Bend the knees, and roll to one side.
4. Pause.
5. Prepare for what's next.

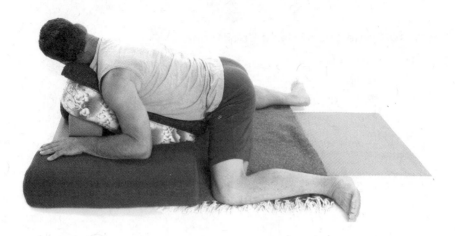

BHEKASANA, VAR. 1 (FROG POSE, VAR. 1)

This variation of Bhekasana is an example of truly bringing the pose to you, by elevating the top end of the bolster and also including a folded blanket on top of the bolster. The adductors shouldn't be screaming. And you may find that even with the smartest method of support, the pose is still uncomfortable. Perhaps it is the general architecture of the pose or a vulnerability that begins to surface. If steady breath and a calm mind cannot be maintained, this pose can be done on the back with the soles of the feet against the wall. Your body will be in the same shape as in the basic pose or its variation, but you will be on your back.

How to Move into Bhekasana, Var. 1

1. Follow the basic pose instructions (page 136) with modified prop placement.
2. Breathe and relax.

How to Come out of Bhekasana, Var. 1

1. Rotate the ankles so that the toes turn under and point toward the tailbone.
2. Push the hands against the floor to straighten the arms, lifting away from the support.
3. Walk the knees behind you, and then sit back into a comfortable position.
4. Pause.
5. Prepare for what's next.

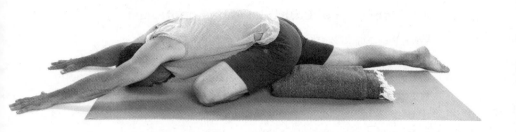

BASIC EKA PADA KAPOTASANA
(ONE-LEGGED PIGEON POSE)

Practicing Basic Eka Pada Kapotasana with support underneath the pelvis can increase the stretch as it lifts the pelvis, which squares itself to the front edge of the mat. This way the body doesn't tilt. If the body tilts to one side while holding the pose, the load may collect around the front knee — not what we want here! The femur (thighbone) of the front leg must externally rotate, and the external rotator muscles must have the flexibility to support the stretch to prevent any load or torque on the knee. This pose isn't for everyone. It can always be practiced on the back in a "figure four" stretch, which is much less risky. If equal flexibility and stability are present in the hip joint, however, it is a pose worth practicing in a prone position. Be ever vigilant of your needs. Refrain from feeding your ego. The risk of injuring a joint isn't worth it.

How to Move into Basic Eka Pada Kapotasana

1. Position a blanket or bolster across the middle of the mat.
2. Kneel just behind the support with your hands slightly ahead of it, and step your left foot over the support.
3. Turn the left thighbone out, and wiggle the left foot toward the right hand while settling the pelvis onto the support.
4. Slowly slide your right leg back, reaching all the way back to straighten the knee, and drop the front of the thigh onto the floor.
5. Stretch the arms forward and rest your head on the floor, or fold your arms to rest the forehead on the top arm.
6. Breathe and relax.

How to Come out of Basic Eka Pada Kapotasana

1. Walk the hands closer to the support.
2. Push the hands against the floor, and turn the back toes under.
3. Lift the right knee off the mat so that you can slide the support out from underneath the pelvis, and roll to the left.
4. Pause.
5. Prepare for the opposite side.

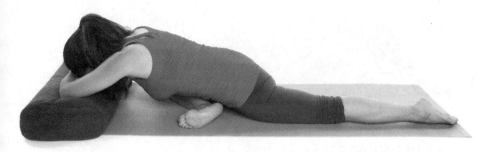

EKA PADA KAPOTASANA, VAR. 1
(ONE-LEGGED PIGEON POSE, VAR. 1)

Variation 1 of Eka Pada Kapotasana reduces the reach of the torso. Once the torso moves below the plane of the hips, as it does in the basic pose, it offers a tremendous stretch to the gluteus (buttocks) and neighboring hip muscles. A bolster or even two bolsters placed underneath the folded arms, to catch the torso, can be enough support to keep you in the pose longer than five breaths. Smile!

How to Move into Eka Pada Kapotasana, Var. 1

1. Follow the basic pose instructions (page 139) with modified prop placement.
2. Breathe and relax.

How to Come out of Eka Pada Kapotasana, Var. 1

Follow the basic pose instructions (page 140).

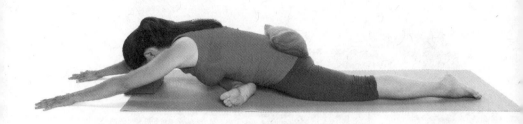

EKA PADA KAPOTASANA, VAR. 2
(ONE-LEGGED PIGEON POSE, VAR. 2)

If you want that extra little something in Eka Pada Kapotasana but are not quite ready to stretch it all out, substitute a block under the forehead for the torso support used in variation 1. I find variation 2 to be great for those who hold tension in the neck while in this pose, an indication that they aren't quite supported enough to let go. Of course, you can always add a 10-pound sandbag across the back pelvis to encourage it to drop into gravity a little more.

How to Move into Eka Pada Kapotasana, Var. 2

1. Follow the basic pose instructions (page 139) with modified prop placement.
2. Breathe and relax.

How to Come out of Eka Pada Kapotasana, Var. 2

Follow the basic pose instructions (page 140).

CHAPTER 8

STILL POSES: FINAL RELAXATION THE YAPANA WAY

....

The way our body relaxes into its Savasana shape tells us much about challenges we may face in other poses.

Savasana (Corpse Pose) is the final pose that all other BEING poses are preparing for. However, when well supported it can also be a pose to begin with that sets the perfect tone for a successful BEING practice. Whether practiced at the beginning, end, or both, Savasana is designed to be experienced as an opportunity to turn away from constant doing, controlling, commanding, and assigning.

There will be times in Savasana when you will feel "relaxation challenged." Sometimes it is because the mind is processing what has come before, or out of nowhere sensations and emotions begin to bubble to the surface. The way our body relaxes into its Savasana shape tells us much about challenges we may face in other poses. Becoming aware of our holding patterns in stillness is just as important as observing them in movement and is a pointer to what kind of support might be necessary to promote more balance overall to our body/mind when practicing Savasana.

In all yoga poses, levels of experience change with time spent in them. You are just as likely to experience such changes in Savasana, even after a complete BEING practice. However, both thoughtful and skillful sequencing of the Yapana BEING and STILL segments will encourage

·the greatest amount of rest with the least amount of effort. And allowing yourself to accept the changes of emotional feelings and physical sensations, as opposite as they may appear, will foster an experience of reconciliation and integration of the two rather than their separation.

Some yoga schools allow for 1 minute of Savasana for every 10 minutes of strong practice. For instance, if you had an asana practice for 60 minutes, the Savasana would be 6 minutes. However, since most Americans spend hardly any time at all deliberately and consciously relaxing, I recommend no less than 10 minutes of Savasana in a 60-minute practice, 15 minutes in a 75-minute practice, and 20 minutes in a 90-minute practice.

Also, you don't have to practice BEING poses before Savasana. In fact, I recommend practicing Savasana every day, with or without BEING poses. Try it for seven straight days, and see what comes. Savasana has strong potential for showing you a doorway into mindfully managing life and promoting feelings of expansion and joy.

HOW WOULD YOU LIKE YOUR SAVASANA?

There are many ways to take rest in Savasana, with or without support. Savasana does not have to be practiced the exact same way every time. Determining the kind of Savasana for the practice is based on what kinds of poses or pranayama were practiced before Savasana. For instance, if the sequence addressed a stiff lower back, a logical choice may be to offer a Savasana that gives support to the lower back. If this is the case, consider practicing Savasana with either the legs elevated or weight on the top thighs to release the lower back into gravity. Or if the sequence focused on opening the chest and shoulders, a logical choice may be to practice a Savasana that includes an eye pillow to support going inside.

SAVASANA AS PREPARATION
FOR A PRANAYAMA PRACTICE

Perhaps you have a pranayama practice toward the end of the asana practice. If so, you may have done poses that focus on opening the front, back, and sides of the waist and the muscles between the chest and shoulders. Practicing a "mini"-Savasana (approximately 3 minutes) is recommended before a pranayama practice. This can help further mentally prepare for pranayama. Of course, after the pranayama practice is completed, a full Savasana is recommended.

General Contraindications for Practicing Savasana

- Pregnancy in the second and third trimesters — elevate the chest so that the heart is higher than the belly

General Benefits of Practicing Savasana

- Encourages one-pointed awareness
- Fosters mental clarity
- Helps to lower blood pressure
- Helps with insomnia
- Reduces fatigue
- Relaxes the body
- Relieves stress

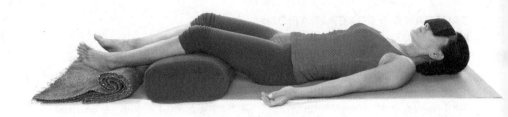

BASIC SAVASANA (CORPSE POSE)

When practicing Savasana, it may take you a few moments to settle into position. Move around a bit to find a good level of comfort, and then commit to where you are. Allow a gentle breath to move in and out, gently rocking your body away from and into gravity.

The simplest of support is shown in the photograph above: a bolster and blanket to support the legs and an eye bag to rest across the eyes.

How to Move into Basic Savasana

1. Rest supine with the legs draped over a bolster, a single- or double-rolled blanket underneath the ankles, and an eye bag resting on the eyes.
2. Rest the arms and hands away from the hips with the palms turned upward.
3. Make a comfortable distance between the shoulders and ears.
4. Relax the skin of the forehead, eyes, and cheeks down toward the bridge of the nose.
5. Deliberately relax the weight of the bones, muscles, organs, fluids, and nerves.
6. Explore and receive the feelings and sensations as they come in and out of your awareness.
7. Experience what it feels like to relax. And relax a little more.

How to Come out of Basic Savasana

1. Allow movement to stir throughout the body.
2. Bend the knees, placing the feet onto the floor.
3. Draw the knees in to the chest, and roll to the right.
4. Pause.
5. Prepare for what's next.

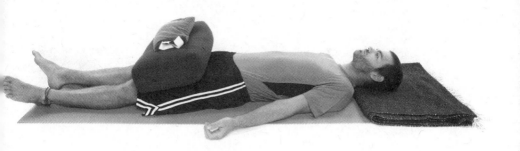

SAVASANA, VAR. 1 (CORPSE POSE, VAR. 1)

Variation 1 of Savasana uses a bolster and a 10-pound sandbag to weigh down the legs and pelvis, which can bring relief to an achy or fatigued lower back.

How to Move into Savasana, Var. 1

1. Follow the basic pose instructions (page 146) with modified prop placement.
2. Breathe and relax.

How to Come out of Savasana, Var. 1

Follow the basic pose instructions (page 146).

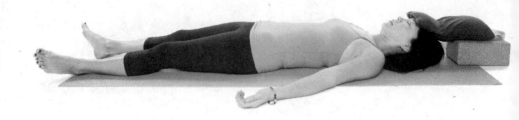

The next two variations (2 and 3) both address tension headaches. Although the causes of tension headaches are still uncertain, researchers believe that most are triggered by internal or environmental stress. Oftentimes the breathing pattern of someone who frequently experiences tension headaches is shallow. Or the breath is held without the person having any awareness of doing so. Poor breathing habits influence our posture and the tension we hold in our body. Variations 2 and 3 both aim to relax the muscles around the face, neck, throat, and shoulders.

SAVASANA, VAR. 2 (CORPSE POSE, VAR. 2)

A block is placed just beyond the top of the head to hold two-thirds of a 10-pound sandbag. The other third of the bag is gently placed across the forehead. The weight of the bag informs the entire skull to relax into gravity.

How to Move into Savasana, Var. 2

1. Follow the basic pose instructions (page 146) with modified prop placement.
2. Breathe and relax.

How to Come out of Savasana, Var. 2

Follow the basic pose instructions (page 146).

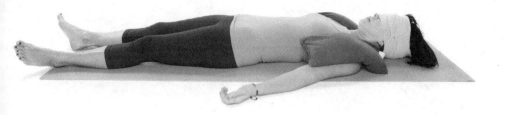

SAVASANA, VAR. 3 (CORPSE POSE, VAR. 3)

Habitual holding of the upper back and neck, along with eyestrain, may trigger tension headaches.

In variation 3 of Savasana, an eye wrap is placed around the head to cover the forehead, ears, and eyes. This soft compression around the skull feels comforting and creates a quiet cocoon refuge from the busyness of the external world. Sandbags on the shoulders weigh them down so that the upper trapeziuses (the large back muscles that extend from the base of the skull to the lower mid back and across the shoulder blades) and levatores scapulae (the muscles that rest on the back and side of the neck) can relax, helping the head, neck, and shoulders to melt away accumulated stress held there.

How to Move into Savasana, Var. 3

1. Follow the basic pose instructions (page 146) with modified prop placement.
2. Breathe and relax.

How to Come out of Savasana, Var. 3

Follow the basic pose instructions (page 146).

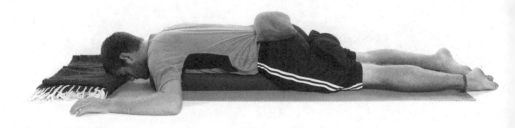

SAVASANA, VAR. 4 (CORPSE POSE, VAR. 4)

This downward-facing variation of Savasana is an interesting option for someone who may want to explore relaxation around the abdominal region. The torso is supported on a bolster with the pubis bone waterfalling off one short end of the bolster. Because not everyone is comfortable resting on the front side of the body, a 10-pound sandbag can be placed across the back of the pelvis and another one across the upper back thighs to settle the pelvis into a neutral position. If necessary, a blanket is placed underneath the head to keep it on the same plane as the spine.

How to Move into Savasana, Var. 4

1. Position a bolster on the mat in a parallel orientation and a blanket on the floor in front of the mat.
2. Lie facedown so the pubis bone is just hanging off the back end of the bolster.
3. Rest the forehead on the blanket.
4. Bring the arms into a goalpost position.
5. Relax and breathe.

How to Come out of Savasana, Var. 4

1. Bend the left knee alongside the bolster.
2. Push the left hand against the floor.
3. Roll to the right side.
4. Pause.
5. Prepare for what's next.

CHAPTER 9

BEING AND BREATHING: THE YAPANA WAY TO MINDFULNESS

A mindfulness practice establishes an inner silence that creates a stress-free environment used to handle a stressful outer environment.

Our world is fast-paced, both internally and externally, but we do have the means to address the chaos. Science has proved that meditation sharpens the mind and produces benefits for everyone. Meditation creates change in brain waves, particularly alpha waves, which are associated with relaxation.

Many people say they don't have the time to devote an hour a day to meditation. Each of us, however, has 10 or 15 minutes for being and breathing, which can open the door to mindfulness or a formal meditation practice. Like most things we learn, there is no way to get good at it other than by doing it.

The word *meditation* can stir up images in our mind — from the old loin-clothed yogi sitting on a mountain to a monk who has taken a vow of silence and hasn't spoken in years or a scantily clad popular yoga teacher posing on the cover of a yoga magazine. I think of meditation as practicing mindfulness and an opportunity to "be" and breathe mindfully. Mindfulness is a time to observe without judgment and take to heart what's present without pushing against or away from your self. A mindfulness practice establishes an inner silence that creates a stress-free environment used to handle a stressful outer environment.

Personal freedom can be yours. You only need to make the investment — in yourself.

There is no right or wrong way to meditate. It can be practiced while sitting, walking, or eating or in any other situation and time you choose. For many who sit while meditating, having a comfortable seat is the biggest challenge. Following are four ways to support your "seat."

General Contraindications for Meditation

- None, other than avoiding long periods of sitting for those with serious back injuries

General Benefits of Meditation

- Fosters mental clarity
- Helps lower blood pressure
- Helps reduce anxiety
- Promotes feelings of steadiness and joy
- Builds self-confidence
- Harmonizes body, mind, and spirit

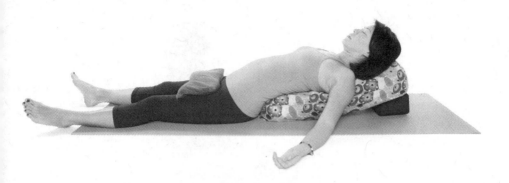

SUPPORTED RECLINING POSE

If you prefer to rest in a reclining position for mindfulness, Supported Reclining Pose keeps the belly, ribs, and chest open and accessible for breathing. This is more often considered a "classical" position for pranayama; however, it can be used for simple mindfulness practices. Or you may practice a basic breathing technique: Belly, Ribs, and Chest breathing (see instructions on page 161).

How to Move into Supported Reclining Pose

1. Position a bolster on the mat in a parallel orientation with a block underneath the top end of the bolster.
2. With your pelvis on the floor and the small of the back against the bottom end of the bolster, lie back, resting the entire remainder of your torso on the bolster.
3. Allow your arms to rest away from the hips with the palms turned upward.
4. Let the legs separate and relax.
5. If you like, place a 10-pound sandbag on the top thighs.
6. Breathe and relax.

How to Come out of Supported Reclining Pose

1. Bend the knees, and set the feet onto the floor.
2. Draw the left arm in to the chest.
3. Push off with the feet, and roll to the right side.
4. Pause.
5. Prepare for what's next.

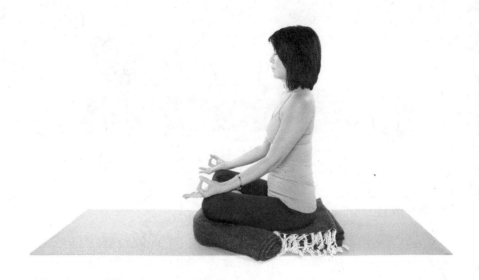

BASIC SEAT FOR MINDFULNESS

A seated position, as opposed to a reclining one, can encourage an alert yet calm approach to practicing mindfulness. One position is not considered better than the other. Practice your preference.

How to Move into Basic Seat for Mindfulness

1. Prepare a folded meditation pad and a long-rolled blanket.
2. Sit upright near the front edge of the meditation pad in a cross-legged position.
3. Wrap the long-rolled blanket around the outer legs, and allow the shins and knees to rest against it.
4. If you like, place the hands in Jnana Mudra, gently touching the thumbs and index fingers together and lightly resting the backs of the hands on the tops of the knees.
5. Be with your breath.
6. Be still.

How to Come out of Basic Seat for Mindfulness

1. Bring your awareness to your whole body by taking a few deep, long inhalations and exhalations.
2. Bring your awareness to the outer corners of your eyes.

3. When you open the eyes, allow the outer corners of the eyes to widen and the eyes themselves to relax toward the back of the sockets — let the landscape come to you rather than reaching with your sight to see it.
4. Straighten the legs.
5. Pause.
6. Prepare for what's next.

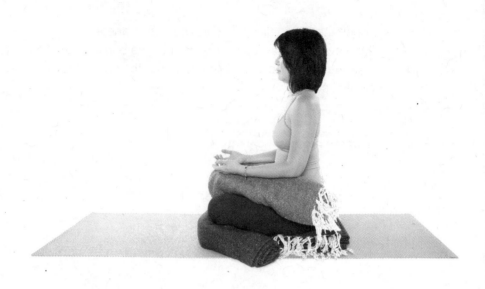

SEAT FOR MINDFULNESS, VAR. 1

Variation 1 of Seat for Mindfulness adds arm support. Play with the position of the hands to find out what position allows the shoulders to remain down and away from the ears, and the head to be balanced on top of the spine. Supporting the lower arms with double-rolled blankets underneath them provides the feedback to relax them even more.

How to Move into Seat for Mindfulness, Var. 1

1. Follow the basic pose instructions (page 154) with modified prop placement.
2. Breathe and relax.

How to Come out of Seat for Mindfulness, Var. 1

Follow the basic pose instructions (page 154).

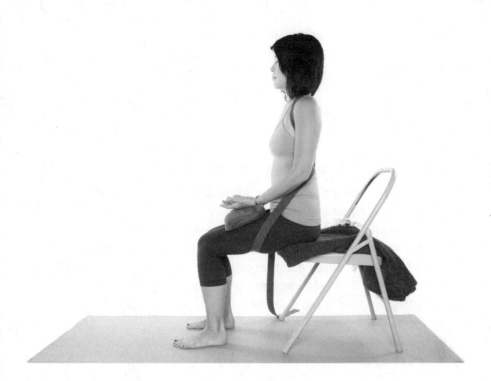

SEAT FOR MINDFULNESS, VAR. 2

Try variation 2 of Seat for Mindfulness if you prefer to sit on a chair. A belt is wrapped around the shoulders and the mid back to draw the shoulders and shoulder blades back and down, and then fastened underneath the legs for lower back support. For this variation, you will need a belt that is at least 8 feet long. A 10-pound sandbag is placed on the top thighs to weigh down the legs, which helps to lengthen the lower back in the upright, seated position.

How to Move into Seat for Mindfulness, Var. 2

1. Place the yoga belt around the back of your neck with the two tails falling equally in front of the body.
2. Bring the tails underneath the armpits and behind the back.
3. Cross one tail over the other, and move both tails to the front of the body.
4. Sit upright on the front edge of a chair with the feet hip distance apart.

5. Fasten the belt underneath the legs.
6. Place a 10-pound sandbag on the top of the thighs.
7. Position the hands with the palms turned upward, and rest them on the sandbag.
8. Be with your breath.
9. Be still.

How to Come out of Seat for Mindfulness, Var. 2

1. Bring your awareness to your whole body by taking a few deep, long inhalations and exhalations.
2. Bring your awareness to the outer corners of your eyes.
3. When you open the eyes, allow the outer corners of the eyes to widen and the eyes themselves to relax toward the back of the sockets — let the landscape come to you rather than reaching with your sight to see it.
4. Release the belt.
5. Pause.
6. Prepare for what's next.

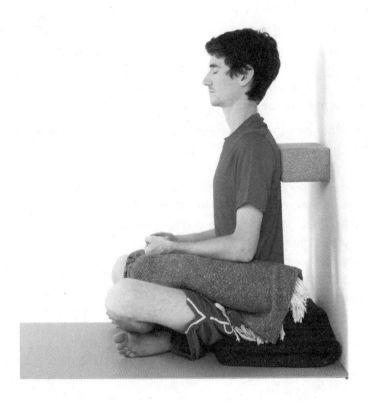

SEAT FOR MINDFULNESS, VAR. 3

Variation 3 of Seat for Mindfulness is an excellent option for someone who tends to collapse in the lower and mid back. It provides both support and feedback to the lower and upper body, including the arms. This is one of my favorite setups for my mindfulness practice. Try it. You may love it.

How to Move into Seat for Mindfulness, Var. 3

1. Position your body near a wall with a meditation pad, two short-rolled blankets, and a block.
2. Place the open-ended edge of the meditation pad next to the wall.
3. Sit upright on the front edge of the meditation pad in a cross-legged position.
4. Place the block on edge against the wall and sit upright against it, so that it supports the shoulder blades.

5. Place a short-rolled blanket underneath each arm for support.
6. Use the feedback of the block to relax the shoulders, lift and broaden the chest, and align the head on top of the spine.

How to Come out of Seat for Mindfulness, Var. 3

1. Bring your awareness to your whole body by taking a few deep, long inhalations and exhalations.
2. Bring your awareness to the outer corners of your eyes.
3. When you open the eyes, allow the outer corners of the eyes to widen and the eyes themselves to relax toward the back of the sockets — let the landscape come to you rather than reaching with your sight to see it.
4. Reach back with a hand to remove the block.
5. Straighten the legs.
6. Pause.
7. Prepare for what's next.

THREE BASIC BREATHING (BASIC PRANAYAMA) TECHNIQUES FOR MINDFULNESS

The following breathing techniques have been around for years. They are not new-and-improved versions. They are an invitation for you to explore, reconcile, and accept what is present or dormant in you simply by being, breathing, and feeling. That is all. Keeping it simple is what these techniques are all about.

Belly, Ribs, and Chest Breathing — Three-Part Breathing

Belly, Ribs, and Chest breathing is a classic introduction to exploring mindfulness via the breath and its relaxation of the body/mind. Yoga practitioners, once introduced to a breath called Ujjayi ("the Victorious Breath"), can be easily entranced by the forced sound of Ujjayi breathing, which is produced by slightly closing the throat at the back of the mouth. As a result, breathing becomes strained, and all sensitive observation of the breath goes out the window. Consider using this simple mindful technique — Belly, Ribs, and Chest breathing — as a way to connect and explore what's happening now. It can be practiced as part of your BEING practice or before it or after it. And it can be practiced in any of the Seats for Mindfulness or the Supported Reclining Pose.

1. In a comfortable seated or supine position, rest the hands lightly across your belly.
2. Bring your interest to the belly, and feel how it gently spreads and settles underneath your hands.
3. Breathe into a soft and merciful belly. There is no right or wrong here, except do not allow the breath to harden the belly as you bring your breath to it. Invite the breath to spread rather than lift the belly. Take your time exploring the breath, and practice accepting all the feelings and sensations that may arise.
4. Slide your hands to lightly rest across the front ribs, and feel how they gently expand and contract underneath your hands.
5. Breathe into this protective structure known as the rib cage. Invite the breath to move the side and back ribs without pushing and forcing the discovery. Take your time exploring the breath, and practice accepting all of the feelings and sensations that may arise.

6. Slide your hands to lightly rest across the chest, and feel how the hands may rise and fall or pull away from each other with each inhalation and exhalation. Explore the chest as two pieces rather than one — as if the right and left sides were two separate parts of the chest. Notice if the breath is stronger on one side than the other. There is nothing to change. Your only interest is in observation and acceptance. Take your time exploring the breath, and practice accepting all the feelings and sensations that may arise.

7. Remove the hands from the chest, and rest them alongside the hips with the palms turned upward.

8. Rest.

Now practice breathing into the three sections in a combined sequence, first bringing your attention to the belly and then gently moving a soft, round, but deep breath up the body, next into the ribs, and finally into the chest. Do not force this. Follow your inhalation from the belly to the ribs and to the chest. Let a long and controlled exhalation release from the belly, ribs, and chest. Pause. Take three normally paced breaths.

1. Practice several rounds without creating hardness in the belly, ribs, chest, throat, or neck.

2. When finished, observe normally paced breaths.

3. Stretch out with your feelings to sense the quality, temperature, and sensations of the breath and your overall experience of what's happening now.

4. Resist nothing, even the concept of resistance.

5. Let your body float in the sensations of its structure, support, and space.

6. When you feel ready to move, draw your interest to the solid floor beneath you.

7. Sense how your body is being moved by the movement of the breath — away from and into gravity.

8. Allow some movement to stir throughout your body.

9. Draw your knees in to the chest.

10. Pause.

11. Roll to the right side.

12. Prepare for what's next.

Center to Periphery Breathing — Breathing Like a Baby

The technique of breathing from the center to the periphery is a balance of directing and following the breath from the navel area (we'll call that your center) outwardly to the space around you (we'll call that the periphery). Have you ever observed a baby breathe? The body moves gently, swaying and rocking as a result of an organic process of each phase of the breath. The Center to Periphery breathing technique gives a gentle massage to the muscles, organs, and tissues that evokes an indescribable calm and steadiness throughout. Ultimately, the goal is to breathe like a baby. Practice Center to Periphery breathing in the Supported Reclining Pose (page 153), as feeling the movement of the breath against the body is easier in a reclining position than in a seated one.

1. Bring your awareness to your center, and notice the breath gently moving you away from gravity on an inhalation and settling you into gravity on an exhalation.
2. Take a few breaths that are a little longer and deeper than usual to help facilitate this.
3. Now relax your skin so that you can perceive the movement the breath has against it and how it plays with the force of gravity.
4. On an inhalation, with the greatest amount of awareness and the least amount of effort, direct your breath from your center to your limbs and into the space around you.
5. On an exhalation, allow the breath to release from the periphery and settle back into your center.
6. Encourage a round, global breath rather than a vertical one, as in Belly, Ribs, and Chest breathing.
7. Follow with two or three normally paced inhalations and exhalations.
8. Continue again with the movement and direction of the breath.
9. When your interest has waned, return to normally paced breathing.
10. Follow the "how to come out" instructions for the Supported Reclining Pose (page 153).

Exchanging Thoughts for Feelings — Breathing and Feeling

The BEING poses provide a safe place to introduce meditation. The Exchanging Thoughts for Feelings breathing technique taps into the deep well of our thoughts and feelings. Exchanging thoughts for feelings is another way to extend and support the life of mindfulness. Because a thought does not want to be looked at for too long, exchanging it for a feeling is a pathway to holding awareness for a longer period of time. My personal preference is to practice this in any of the Seats for Mindfulness, as sitting upright helps to keep me interested in the process.

1. Find your preferred Seat for Mindfulness.
2. Gently place your hands against your chest.
3. Start breathing mindfully.
4. Be aware of the present thought, and exchange it for a feeling.
5. Be with the feeling for as long as you can until another thought wants to enter.
6. Exchange the new thought for a feeling, and continue the cycle until your disinterest is stronger than your ability to hold interest.
7. To complete the process, take three or four deep breaths.
8. Follow the "how to come out" instructions for the Seat for Mindfulness you've chosen (page 154, 156, or 158).

CHAPTER 10

PURPOSEFUL PRACTICES

....

There is real power in being peaceful.

So many of us are living a disconnected life that leaves us feeling constantly busy and "stressed-out." We're spending more time surviving than we're spending living. We've replaced a well-balanced meal with several lattes, and we sit in a chair in front of a computer screen for hours each day. On top of that, we have to manage all of our personal and professional obligations. This accumulation of negative energy creates a wall between our "doing" and "being" selves as opposed to integrating the two. Purposeful Practices are specific sequences that help to remedy a lifestyle that overloads our system — and weakens us physically and physiologically — causing injuries, common ailments, and mental and emotional trauma. Purposeful Practices provide the self-care that is necessary for shedding the stresses accumulated throughout each day.

Individual poses in a sequence can be switched with other poses to make adjustments. However, pose placement in any sequence is important and should not be approached haphazardly. Because each pose has a physiological effect on the body/mind, its position in a sequence can alter the overall benefits of the sequence.

The following sequences are examples of what is possible. They target either specific areas of the body or common challenges. Each one is approximately 30 to 60 minutes long and is designed to achieve a purposeful practice for well-being, break down the wall of stress, and refuel your spiritual self. Each pose is shown in its recommended form, although you may practice any variation to meet your individual needs.

The ideal situation is to practice without any distractions and to have access to all your yoga props. The following are recommendations to further support your journey of self-care:

- The best time to practice is when you can fully tune in and be present. Try scheduling your practice at the same time of the day throughout the week to foster consistency. Whatever time you determine is best, be prepared to give yourself to it whole-heartedly.
- Turn off your phone.
- Practice in a clean and smoke-free environment that provides fresh air and is temperature controlled.
- Have available all the yoga props and a blanket in case you get cold.
- Background music may be used to induce a state of deep re-laxation.

TIME IS ON YOUR SIDE

If you are new to a supported practice, take your time with the props. You'll need some practice to get acquainted with positioning the yoga props so that they provide the right support. Each sequence can be practiced as shown, or you can modify it to meet your personal prefer-ences. It is important, however, to consider the physiological effects that each pose provides. For instance, if you are going for total rest and relax-ation, it makes less sense to practice back bends before the STILL pose, because back bends are more wakeful to the nervous system, whereas forward bends and some inversions are more calming and cooling. The following timetable shows the recommended minutes for different poses. You can use it as a guide to help direct you into the kind of practice you wish to experience.

TIMETABLE: MINUTES SPENT IN POSES

Back Bends	2–5, gradually increase to 15
Twists	3, gradually increase to 10
Forward Bends	2–5, gradually increase to 10
Inversions	3, gradually increase to 20
Lateral Bends	3, gradually increase to 5
Reclining Standing	2–5, gradually increase to 10
Reclining Leg Stretches	3, gradually increase to 5
Shoulder Stretch	3, gradually increase to 5
Prone	3, gradually increase to 5
Final Relaxation	15–20
Seats for Meditation	5, gradually increase to 30

POWERFUL PEACE

At times life can feel overwhelming. This is when we can turn to our practice to receive immediate loving care. Where practice is done, a problem
is solved. A still mind is what ultimately solves a problem. This sequence
is designed to still and quiet the mind and instill a calm and steadiness
throughout. Practice this sequence to combat holiday stress, physical
fatigue, mental exhaustion, or just plain crankiness. It you want to be at
peace, you have to practice being peaceful. If you want to experience
peace around you, you have to practice being peaceful. If you want
others to be peaceful, you have to practice being peaceful around them.

1. Belly, Ribs, and Chest breathing in Basic Reclining Bound Angle
   Pose (page 48)
2. Basic Fish Pose (page 37)
3. Basic Stomach Turn Pose (page 70)
4. Basic Child Pose (page 133)
5. Basic Reclining Bridge Pose (page 44)
6. Basic Seated Forward Bend Pose (page 87)
7. Basic "Legs up the Chair" Pose (page 81)
8. Basic Corpse Pose — 3 minutes (page 146)
9. Exchanging Thoughts for Feelings breathing in Supported Reclining Pose (page 153)
10. Corpse Pose, Var. 3 (page 149)

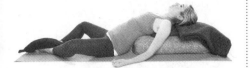

1. BASIC RECLINING BOUND ANGLE POSE

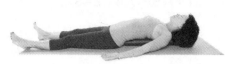

2. BASIC FISH POSE

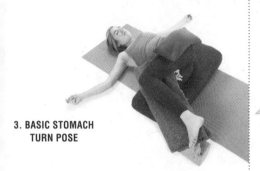

3. BASIC STOMACH TURN POSE

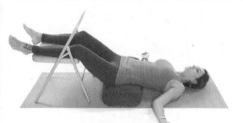

4. BASIC CHILD POSE

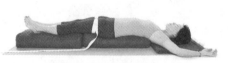

5. BASIC RECLINING BRIDGE POSE

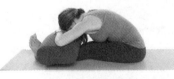

6. BASIC SEATED FORWARD BEND POSE

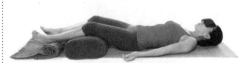

7. BASIC "LEGS UP THE CHAIR" POSE

8. BASIC CORPSE POSE — 3 MINUTES

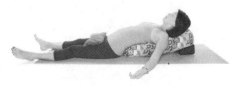

9. SUPPORTED RECLINING POSE

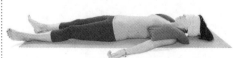

10. CORPSE POSE, VAR. 3

STIFF SHOULDERS

Many factors make up a healthy posture, and the shoulders play a key role. A slouched posture with rounded shoulders overstretches and strains the upper back and neck and weakens the muscles between the shoulder blades. Habitual slouching collapses the chest, compresses the thoracic diaphragm, and can develop into stress injuries or dysfunction in your shoulder joints. Ouch!

This sequence focuses on releasing neck and shoulder tension while supporting and stretching neighboring muscles. It's the ultimate reversal for slouched shoulders and for someone who spends a lot of time sitting at the computer.

1. Reclining Shoulder Stretch (page 131)
2. Side-Lying Stretch Pose, Var. 2 (page 106)
3. Reclining Revolved Triangle Pose, Var. 1 (page 65)
4. Basic Camel Pose (page 51)
5. Stomach Turn Pose, Var. 1 (page 72)
6. Basic Reclining Bridge Pose (page 44)
7. Basic Child Pose (page 133)
8. Corpse Pose, Var. 3 (page 149)

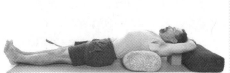

1. RECLINING SHOULDER STRETCH

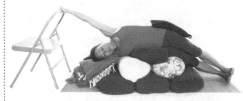

2. SIDE-LYING STRETCH POSE, VAR. 2

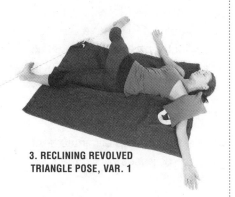

3. RECLINING REVOLVED TRIANGLE POSE, VAR. 1

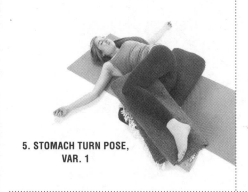

4. BASIC CAMEL POSE

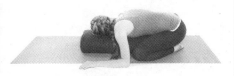

5. STOMACH TURN POSE, VAR. 1

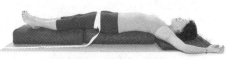

6. BASIC RECLINING BRIDGE POSE

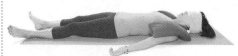

7. BASIC CHILD POSE

8. CORPSE POSE, VAR. 3

LOWER BACK LUCK

Millions of Americans complain of lower backaches when there is nothing structurally wrong. Perhaps you strained your back lifting something or working out or simply used poor biomechanics throughout the day to perform daily activities. Maybe you spend most of your day sitting at a computer — our bodies were not built for that. Of course, accumulated stress can settle in your back without your even knowing it.

There are several processes for healing an achy lower back. First, ease the mind with simple breathing exercises. Studies show that a calm approach to any physical challenge can help foster positive results. Next, determine the other processes that are needed to promote healing. Your condition may require traction, mobility, stability, flexibility, or any combination of those.

This sequence encourages flexibility and traction to help eliminate tightness and compression. Follow the sequence of poses recommended, and turn an achy lower back into lower back luck!

1. Basic Child Pose (page 133)
2. Basic Half Knee to Chest Pose (page 117)
3. Reclining Big Toe 1 Pose, Var. 1 (page 122)
4. Fish Pose, Var. 2 (page 39)
5. Revolved Knee Squeeze Pose, Var. 2 (page 69)
6. Half Knee to Chest Pose, Var. 1 (page 118)
7. Basic Seated Forward Bend Pose (page 87)
8. Basic "Legs up the Chair" Pose (page 81)
9. "Legs up the Chair" Pose, Var. 1 (page 83)
10. Corpse Pose, Var. 1 (page 147)

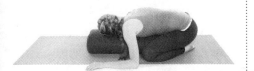

1. BASIC CHILD POSE

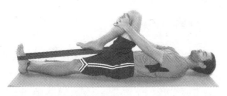

2. BASIC HALF KNEE TO CHEST POSE

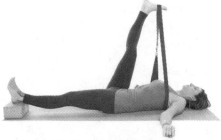

3. RECLINING BIG TOE 1 POSE, VAR. 1

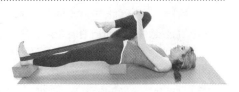

4. FISH POSE, VAR. 2

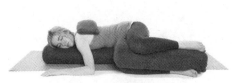

5. REVOLVED KNEE SQUEEZE POSE, VAR. 2

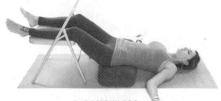

6. HALF KNEE TO CHEST POSE, VAR. 1

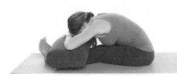

**7. BASIC SEATED
FORWARD BEND POSE**

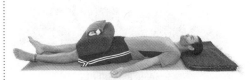

**8. BASIC "LEGS
UP THE CHAIR" POSE**

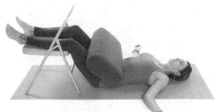

**9. "LEGS UP THE CHAIR" POSE,
VAR. 1**

10. CORPSE POSE, VAR. 1

HAPPY HIPSTERS

Do you need to unlock your hips? Many people have tight hip flexors (muscles that run down the front of the hip joints). Hours of sitting keep the hips in a flexed position that contracts these muscles. Hip flexors allow for forward leg movement and upward knee drive, needed in most athletics. Strategic placement of yoga props will support the hips while gently using gravity in a friendly manner to stretch muscles and connective tissue. This sequence is composed of seated and reclining poses and will improve your hip flexibility and mobility.

1. Basic Reclining Bound Angle Pose (page 48)
2. Basic Reclining Extended Triangle Pose (page 108)
3. Reclining Warrior 2 Pose, Var. 1 (page 114)
4. Revolved Head to Knee Pose, Var. 1 (page 100)
5. One-Legged Pigeon Pose, Var. 2 (page 142)
6. Stomach Turn Pose, Var. 2 (page 73)
7. Reclining Big Toe 1 Pose, Var. 1 (page 122)
8. Basic Reclining Big Toe 2 Pose (page 124)
9. Reclining Revolved Big Toe Pose, Var. 1 (page 129)
10. Basic Child Pose (page 133)
11. Basic "Legs up the Chair" Pose (page 81)
12. Basic Corpse Pose (page 146)

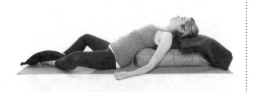

**1. BASIC RECLINING
BOUND ANGLE POSE**

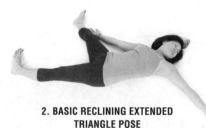

**2. BASIC RECLINING EXTENDED
TRIANGLE POSE**

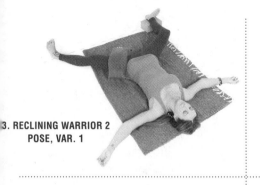

3. RECLINING WARRIOR 2
POSE, VAR. 1

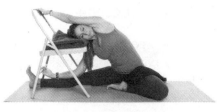

4. REVOLVED HEAD TO KNEE POSE,
VAR. 1

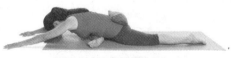

5. ONE-LEGGED PIGEON POSE, VAR. 2

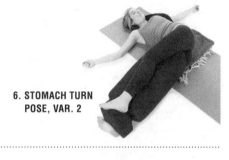

6. STOMACH TURN
POSE, VAR. 2

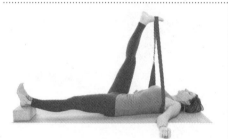

7. RECLINING BIG TOE 1 POSE, VAR. 1

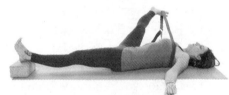

8. BASIC RECLINING BIG TOE 2 POSE

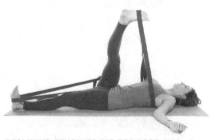

9. RECLINING REVOLVED BIG TOE POSE, VAR. 1

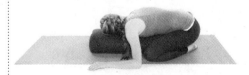

10. BASIC CHILD POSE

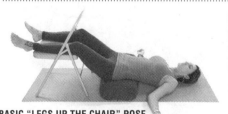

11. BASIC "LEGS UP THE CHAIR" POSE

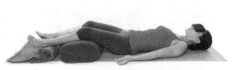

12. BASIC CORPSE POSE

ACTIVE RECOVERY FOR ATHLETES

All the weekend warriors, this sequence is for you! Having worked with many professional athletes, I understand the need for active recovery from demanding workouts. Athletes may suffer from muscle soreness and imbalances from overworked muscles, which can result in shortened and tight muscles. An intelligent Yapana BEING practice is a wise approach to repairing these muscles. The following sequence focuses on stretching large muscle groups that are overloaded from repetitive movements, running, cycling, golf, and sports of all kinds.

1. Basic Fish Pose (page 37)
2. Reclining Bound Angle Pose, Var. 2 (page 50)
3. Basic Reclining Extended Triangle Pose (page 108)
4. Basic Reclining Warrior 2 Pose (page 112)
5. Basic Reclining Revolved Triangle Pose (page 63)
6. Camel Pose, Var. 2 (page 54)
7. Stomach Turn Pose, Var. 1 (page 72)
8. Child Pose, Var. 1 (page 134)
9. Basic Half Knee to Chest Pose (page 117)
10. Reclining Big Toe 1 Pose, Var. 2 (page 123)
11. Seated Wide-Angle Pose, Var. 2 (page 96)
12. Basic Corpse Pose — 3 minutes (page 146)
13. Center to Periphery breathing in Supported Reclining Pose (page 153)
14. Basic Corpse Pose (page 146)

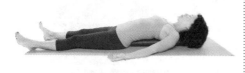

1. BASIC FISH POSE

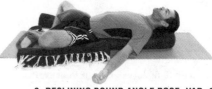

2. RECLINING BOUND ANGLE POSE, VAR. 2

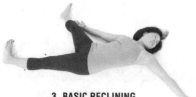

3. BASIC RECLINING EXTENDED TRIANGLE POSE

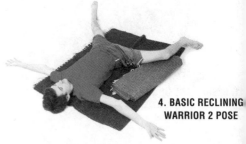

4. BASIC RECLINING WARRIOR 2 POSE

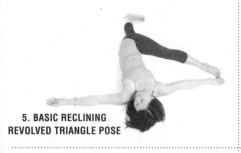

5. BASIC RECLINING REVOLVED TRIANGLE POSE

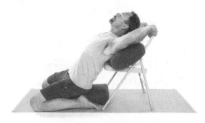

6. CAMEL POSE, VAR. 2

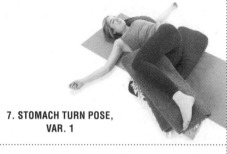

7. STOMACH TURN POSE, VAR. 1

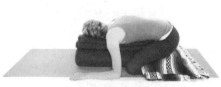

8. CHILD POSE, VAR. 1

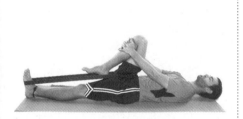

9. BASIC HALF KNEE TO CHEST POSE

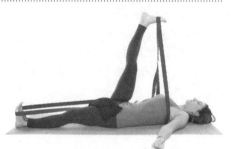

10. RECLINING BIG TOE 1 POSE, VAR. 2

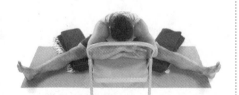

11. SEATED WIDE-ANGLE POSE, VAR. 2

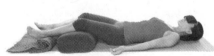

12. BASIC CORPSE POSE — 3 MINUTES

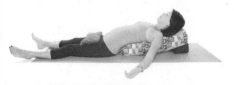

13. SUPPORTED RECLINING POSE

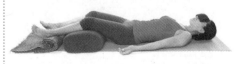

14. BASIC CORPSE POSE

TENSION TAMER

Posture can affect respiration and blood circulation to the brain, causing muscle tension that may result in a tension headache. Although a yoga practice cannot take credit for eliminating a tension headache, an intelligent Yapana BEING practice — focused on correcting poor postural habits, lengthening the neck, shoulder, and back muscles — goes a long way toward reducing the potential for an impending headache caused by the shortening of these muscles.

1. Exchanging Thoughts for Feelings breathing in Corpse Pose, Var. 2 (page 148)
2. Basic Side-Lying Stretch Pose (page 103)
3. Fish Pose, Var. 1 (page 38)
4. Basic Camel Pose (page 51)
5. Basic Revolved Knee Squeeze Pose (page 66)
6. Basic "Legs up the Chair" Pose (page 81)
7. Basic Reclining Bridge Pose (page 44)
8. Seated Wide-Angle Pose, Var. 1 (page 95)
9. Basic Seated Forward Bend Pose (page 87)
10. Corpse Pose, Var. 3 (page 149)

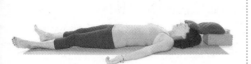

1. CORPSE POSE, VAR. 2

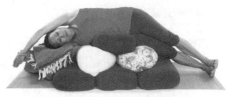

2. BASIC SIDE-LYING STRETCH POSE

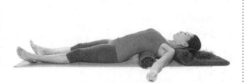

3. FISH POSE, VAR. 1

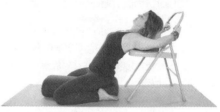

4. BASIC CAMEL POSE

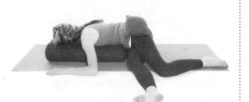

5. BASIC REVOLVED KNEE
SQUEEZE POSE

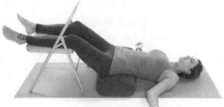

6. BASIC "LEGS
UP THE CHAIR" POSE

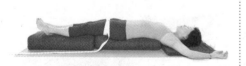

7. BASIC RECLINING BRIDGE POSE

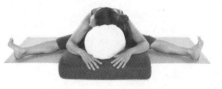

8. SEATED WIDE-ANGLE POSE, VAR. 1

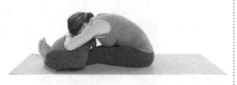

9. BASIC SEATED FORWARD BEND POSE

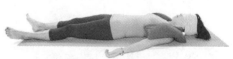

10. CORPSE POSE, VAR. 3

IMMUNITY ENHANCER

The adrenal glands are responsible for releasing hormones in response to stress. When the body is in constant stress mode, these glands work overtime and put strain on the immune system. This sequence focuses on preventing the adrenals from firing. I also recommend that you laugh more! Laughter stimulates circulation and aids in muscle relaxation, both of which help reduce some symptoms of stress and boost immunity.

1. Basic "Legs up the Chair" Pose (page 81)
2. Basic Reclining Bound Angle Pose (page 48)
3. Reclining Bridge Pose, Var. 1 (page 45)
4. Reclining Bridge Pose, Var. 2 (page 46)
5. Reclining Bridge Pose, Var. 3 (page 47)
6. Basic Frog Pose (page 136)
7. Revolved Knee Squeeze Pose, Var. 1 (page 68)
8. Basic "Legs up the Wall" Pose (page 77)
9. Basic Seated Forward Bend Pose (page 87)
10. Basic Child Pose (page 133)
11. Basic Corpse Pose — 3 minutes (page 146)
12. Any mindfulness practice in Supported Reclining Pose (page 153)
13. Basic Corpse Pose (page 146)

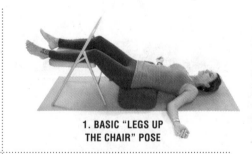

1. BASIC "LEGS UP THE CHAIR" POSE

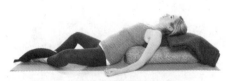

2. BASIC RECLINING BOUND ANGLE POSE

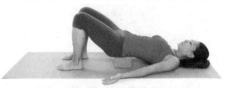

3. RECLINING BRIDGE POSE, VAR. 1

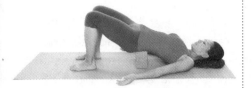

4. RECLINING BRIDGE POSE, VAR. 2

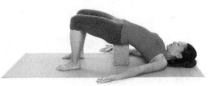

5. RECLINING BRIDGE POSE, VAR. 3

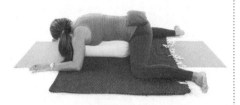

6. BASIC FROG POSE

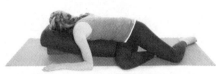

7. REVOLVED KNEE SQUEEZE POSE, VAR. 1

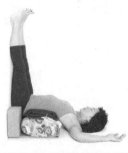

8. BASIC "LEGS UP THE WALL" POSE

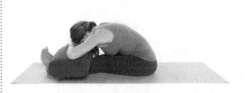

9. BASIC SEATED FORWARD BEND POSE

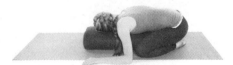

10. BASIC CHILD POSE

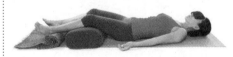

11. BASIC CORPSE POSE — 3 MINUTES

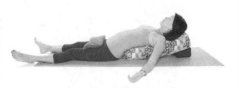

12. SUPPORTED RECLINING POSE

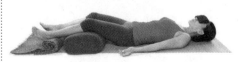

13. BASIC CORPSE POSE

PMS RELIEF

The cycles of a woman's body are both beautiful and complex. A dedicated yoga practice that includes a Yapana BEING practice supports managing the cycles with greater ease. A woman's cycles are a delicate balance of menstruation, pregnancy, and menopause. This Yapana BEING sequence supports menstruation; the next one, "Menopause Makeover," supports menopause; and chapter 11 offers a detailed sequence for pregnancy.

The symptoms of premenstrual syndrome (PMS) include bloating, cramping, muscle tenderness, joint aches, headache, fatigue, tension, anxiety, and mood swings. Thankfully, women typically don't experience all the listed symptoms at once. This Yapana BEING sequence is a complete practice that can help to decrease or even eliminate PMS symptoms.

1. Basic Child Pose (page 133)
2. Basic Reclining Bound Angle Pose (page 48)
3. Fish Pose, Var. 1 (page 38)
4. Basic Reclining Big Toe 1 Pose (page 120)
5. Reclining Big Toe 2 Pose, Var. 1 (page 126)
6. Reclining Revolved Big Toe Pose, Var. 1 (page 129)
7. Seated Wide-Angle Pose, Var. 1 (page 95)
8. Reclining Bridge Pose, Var. 1 (page 45)
9. "Legs up the Chair" Pose, Var. 1 (page 83)
10. Basic Corpse Pose (page 146)

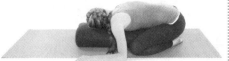

1. BASIC CHILD POSE

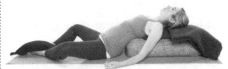

2. BASIC RECLINING BOUND ANGLE POSE

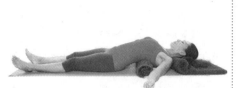

3. FISH POSE, VAR. 1

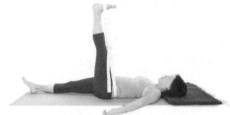

4. BASIC RECLINING BIG TOE 1 POSE

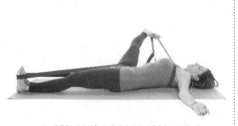

5. RECLINING BIG TOE 2 POSE, VAR. 1

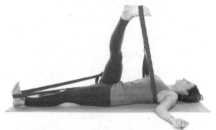

6. RECLINING REVOLVED BIG TOE POSE, VAR. 1

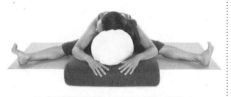

7. SEATED WIDE-ANGLE POSE, VAR. 1

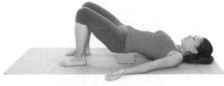

8. RECLINING BRIDGE POSE, VAR. 1

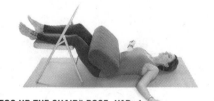

9. "LEGS UP THE CHAIR" POSE, VAR. 1

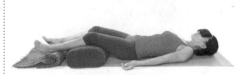

10. BASIC CORPSE POSE

MENOPAUSE MAKEOVER

Menopause symptoms include hot flashes, night sweats, forgetfulness, insomnia, mood changes, and weight gain, any of which can range from irritating to debilitating. This sequence focuses on poses that help to cool the nervous system and calm your nerves. Basic Inverted Two-Legged Staff Pose is the most energetic pose I've included. It provides a nice opening for the back, shoulders, and front thighs, and I enjoy it as part of this sequence. The practice is meant to support you. If any of the poses feel agitating, skip them. Ultimately, allow your symptoms to guide your approach. Each day we bring a different body, mind, and breath to the practice. This Yapana BEING practice promotes self-reflection and the kind of mind that quietly sits up, fostering a level of awareness that supports and directs a healthy attitude needed to face these changing times.

1. Basic "Legs up the Wall" Pose (page 77)
2. Basic Reclining Bound Angle Pose (page 48)
3. Basic Reclining Extended Triangle Pose (page 108)
4. Basic Revolved Head to Knee Pose (page 98)
5. Basic Inverted Two-Legged Staff Pose (page 55)
6. Reclining Bridge Pose, Var. 1 (page 45)
7. Reclining Bridge Pose, Var. 2 (page 46)
8. Reclining Bridge Pose, Var. 3 (page 47)
9. Basic Child Pose (page 133)
10. Basic Seated Forward Bend Pose (page 87)
11. Basic Seated Wide-Angle Pose (page 93)
12. Basic Corpse Pose (page 146)

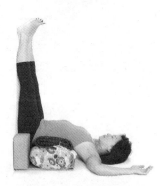

1. BASIC "LEGS UP THE WALL" POSE

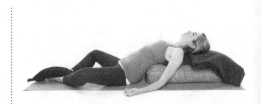

2. BASIC RECLINING BOUND ANGLE POSE

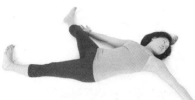

3. BASIC RECLINING EXTENDED
TRIANGLE POSE

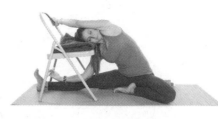

4. BASIC REVOLVED HEAD TO KNEE POSE

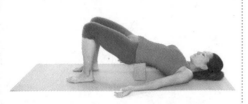

5. BASIC INVERTED TWO-LEGGED STAFF POSE

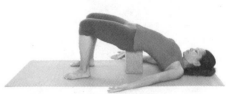

6. RECLINING BRIDGE POSE, VAR. 1

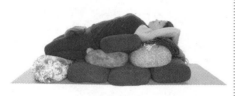

7. RECLINING BRIDGE POSE, VAR. 2

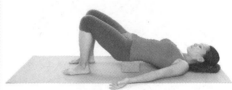

8. RECLINING BRIDGE POSE, VAR. 3

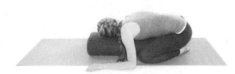

9. BASIC CHILD POSE

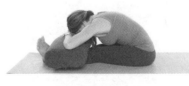

10. BASIC SEATED FORWARD BEND POSE

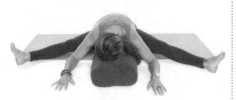

11. BASIC SEATED WIDE-ANGLE POSE

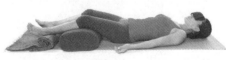

12. BASIC CORPSE POSE

CHAPTER 11

PRENATAL PRACTICE

....

The right prop support can teach the skill necessary for experiencing a balanced approach for doing, being, and breathing in a yoga pose.

A Yapana BEING practice can serve as a healthy strategy to manage and relieve common discomforts that pregnancy may bring. It also prepares you for labor and delivery — physically, mentally, and spiritually. If you are new to a restorative yoga practice, there is no better time to begin one than at the start of your pregnancy. The gentle and therapeutic nature of this practice is the perfect combination for reducing tension and emotional stress and for creating optimal health and a positive childbirth experience for you and your baby.

Pay attention to what you feel in each pose of the sequence, and as with any other yoga practice, trust your instincts and honor your body's needs. Western medical professionals consider the first trimester to be the highest risk for miscarriage and the period in which you experience the most changes. Be extra gentle with yourself. There is no need to push the stretches. Rather, relaxation is most important. Throughout your pregnancy, but especially from halfway through it to the end, keep the heart higher than the pelvis in any reclining position. This ensures that the weight of your uterus doesn't compress the vena cava, a major blood vessel that is responsible for blood flow to your baby. Because this blood vessel is located to the right of your spine, some doctors recommend resting on your left side to allow blood to flow more freely to your baby.

Therefore, when exiting any of the poses described in this chapter, the instructions will direct you to roll to the left side. In the last trimester, consider doing a Yapana BEING practice each day, whether it is for 30 minutes or 90. It will help to strengthen your coping mechanisms, which will come in very handy during labor!

I practiced yoga throughout all three of my pregnancies. Some days I felt like moving, while other days I wanted to practice only Reclining Bound Angle Pose or "Legs up the Wall." My needs changed, as each pregnancy was different. I leaned on my practice when I needed to be held up, slowed down, or kept present. It empowered me as a woman, and I would be forever transformed by what was to come.

You may practice all kinds of yoga styles and make modifications to suit your growing needs. The poses presented in this chapter are meant to be performed as a sequence, one that's similar to the Powerful Peace sequence. Do this Prenatal Practice sequence when you want some serious R&R and desire to deeply connect with your baby.

General Contraindications for Practicing Yoga during Pregnancy

- As with all exercise and stretching, be sure to have your doctor's permission before continuing your yoga practice.

General Benefits of Practicing Yoga during Pregnancy

- Establishes conscious breathing, which is good for managing stress levels and high blood pressure
- Promotes stretching, which keeps your body limber for the delivery
- Fosters a quiet connection with your baby

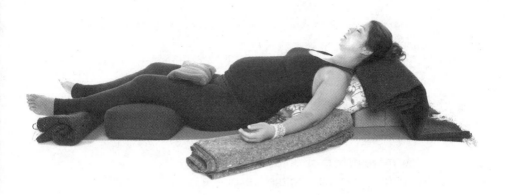

SAVASANA, PRENATAL VAR.
(CORPSE POSE, PRENATAL VAR.)

How to Move into Savasana, Prenatal Var.

1. Position two bolsters on the mat — one parallel and approximately a third of the way from the top end of the mat with two blocks placed underneath the top end of the bolster, and the other perpendicular to the mat near its bottom end.
2. Place a long-rolled blanket at the bottom end of the mat for ankle support.
3. Place a Foundation or a double-folded blanket across the top end of the bolster that's parallel to the mat.
4. Position accordion-folded blankets on either side of the bolster to be used as arm support.
5. Have a sandbag nearby.
6. Sit on the mat so that the bottom edge of the bolster parallel to the mat is against the sacrum, so that when you lie back on the bolster in a supine position, its bottom edge is underneath the lower back. Drape the legs over the bolster at the bottom end of the mat, positioning the ankles on the long-rolled blanket.
7. If you like, place a sandbag on the top thighs to weigh down the legs and pelvis.
8. Rest the arms and hands on the accordion-folded blankets.
9. Create a comfortable distance between the shoulders and ears.
10. Relax the skin of the forehead, eyes, and cheeks down toward the bridge of the nose.

11. Deliberately relax the weight of the bones, muscle, organs, fluids, and nerves.
12. Explore and receive the feelings and sensations as they come in and out of your awareness.
13. Experience what it feels like to relax. And relax a little more.

How to Come out of Savasana, Prenatal Var.

1. Allow movement to stir throughout the body.
2. Bend the knees, placing the feet on the floor.
3. Draw the right arm in to the chest.
4. Push the feet against the floor, and roll to the left.

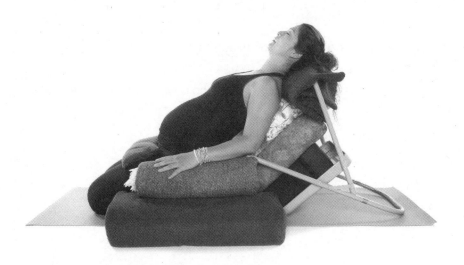

SUPTA VIRASANA, PRENATAL VAR.
(RECLINING HERO POSE, PRENATAL VAR.)

How to Move into Supta Virasana, Prenatal Var.

1. Position a sturdy folding chair upside down at the top end of the mat.
2. Place two or three blocks on the underside of the chair seat.
3. Stack two bolsters lengthwise on top of the blocks.
4. Cover the top, back rung of the chair with a blanket.
5. Position two bolsters on either side of the chair and a short-rolled blanket on top of each bolster, to be used for arm support.
6. Facing away from the support, kneel in front of it and use the hands to stretch the calf muscles away from the knees and toward the heels.
7. Place the hands on the feet to use the arms as leverage to lift the chest and safely lie back onto the bolster, resting the head on the blanket covering the rung and resting the arms on their supports.
8. If you like, place a sandbag on top of the upper thighs to weigh down the legs and pelvis.
9. Lift and broaden the chest.
10. Breathe and relax.

How to Come out of Supta Virasana, Prenatal Var.

1. Gently tuck the chin.
2. Push the hands against the feet or the floor to use as leverage to lift up and out of the pose.
3. Pause.
4. Prepare for what's next.

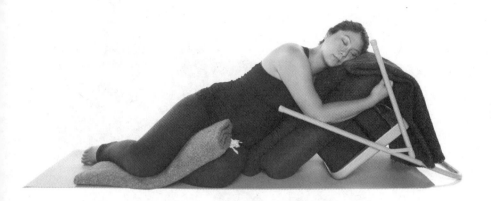

PARIVRTTA PAVANMUKTASANA, PRENATAL VAR.
(REVOLVED KNEE SQUEEZE POSE, PRENATAL VAR.)

How to Move into Parivrtta Pavanmuktasana, Prenatal Var.

1. Use the same setup as in Supta Virasana, Prenatal Var. (page 191), but replace the top bolster with a blanket.
2. Have a long-folded blanket available for the legs.
3. Sit with the left hip against the short end of the bolster, and bend both legs behind you in a soft 90° position. Place the long-folded blanket between the legs.
4. Place your hands on the floor at either side of the bolster, and push them against the floor as leverage to lift the chest and rotate it to the left, but keep the head turned in the same direction as the knees.
5. Lower the torso onto the bolster.
6. Position the arms slightly inward under the top end of the bolster.
7. Breathe and relax.

How to Come out of Parivrtta Pavanmuktasana, Prenatal Var.

1. Keep the chin in a neutral position relative to a neutral skull.
2. Place the hands on the floor underneath the shoulders.
3. Push the hands against the floor to straighten the arms and lift the torso away from the bolster.
4. Straighten both legs, and sit upright.
5. Pause.
6. Prepare for the opposite side.

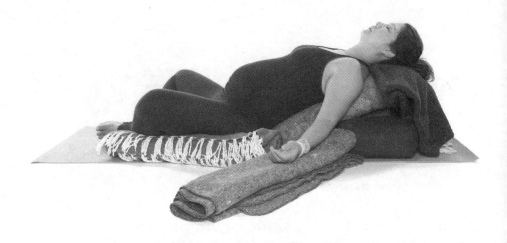

SUPTA BADDHA KONASANA, PRENATAL VAR.
(RECLINING BOUND ANGLE POSE, PRENATAL VAR.)

How to Move into Supta Baddha Konasana, Prenatal Var.

1. Position one bolster on your mat in a parallel orientation. Place two blocks on the top end of the bolster, and another bolster on top, with the blocks lifting the top end of the top bolster.
2. Place a Foundation folded blanket on the top end of the top bolster.
3. Position accordion double-folded blankets on either side of the bolster to be used as arm support.
4. Position long-rolled blankets almost parallel to the sides of the mat to be used as leg support.
5. Sit in front of the short end of the bolster, and bring the soles of the feet together so the knees and thighs fall to the sides and rest on the long-rolled blankets.
6. Using your hands for leverage, gently lie back onto the support.
7. Allow the lower body to relax and sink into the floor and the upper body to open.
8. Breathe and relax.

How to Come out of Supta Baddha Konasana, Prenatal Var.

1. Gently tuck the chin.
2. Use the hands as leverage against the floor to lift up and out of the pose.
3. Slide one foot out to the side and then straighten the leg, followed by the other leg.
4. Pause with the legs straight, and sit upright.
5. Prepare for what's next.

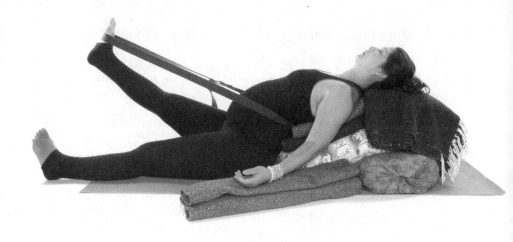

SUPTA PADANGUSTHASANA 1, PRENATAL VAR. (RECLINING BIG TOE 1 POSE, PRENATAL VAR.)

How to Move into Supta Padangusthasana 1, Prenatal Var.

1. Fasten a yoga belt into a loop a little longer than the length of the entire leg, and have it nearby.
2. Position a bolster at the top end of your mat in a perpendicular orientation. Place another bolster on top of the first one, so that the first bolster props up the head end of the second bolster.
3. Place two double-folded blankets on the top bolster, stair-stepped (with a 2-inch distance between the bottom edges of the blankets).
4. Lie back on the bolster, place the belt around the middle back and the sole of the right foot, and extend the right leg as high as you comfortably can.
5. Stretch the left leg out in front of you.
6. Relax the arms on their supports with the palms turned upward.
7. Breathe and relax.

How to Come out of Supta Padangusthasana, Prenatal Var.

1. Bend the right leg, and place the foot on the floor.
2. Bend the bottom leg, and place the foot on the floor.
3. Pause.
4. Prepare for the opposite side, shifting the belt to the left foot.
5. When both legs have been stretched, bend the knees, keeping the feet as wide as the mat, and use the hands against the floor to push yourself to an upright seated position.
6. Pause.
7. Prepare for the opposite side.

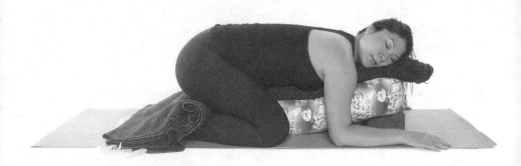

BALASANA, PRENATAL VAR.
(CHILD POSE, PRENATAL VAR.)

How to Move into Balasana, Prenatal Var.

1. Start in a table position on hands and knees, resting on the tops of the feet.
2. Position the legs wide enough to rest outside your side ribs, and slide a bolster between the legs.
3. Bend at the hips to bring the pelvis down to the heel bones, and rest the torso on the bolster.
4. Turn the head to the right, so that the right nostril is on top.
5. Rest the arms in a goalpost position.
6. If the hips do not reach the heels, place a double-folded blanket between the hips and heels to fill the space.

How to Come out of Balasana, Prenatal Var.

1. Keep the chin in a neutral position relative to a neutral skull.
2. Turn the head to rest the forehead on the bolster.
3. Place the hands on the floor underneath the shoulders, and straighten the arms to lift the torso away from the bolster.
4. Sit back on the heels or in any comfortable position.
5. Pause.
6. Prepare for what's next.

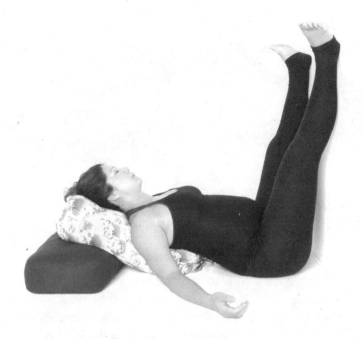

VIPARITA KARANI, PRENATAL VAR.
("LEGS UP THE WALL" POSE, PRENATAL VAR.)

How to Move into Viparita Karani, Prenatal Var.

1. Position two bolsters near a wall, the first bolster perpendicular to the wall with its bottom edge approximately 2 feet away from a wall and the other bolster parallel to the wall and underneath the top half of the first bolster so that they form a T shape.
2. Lie down against the inclined bolster with the pelvis near the wall and the legs up the wall.
3. Bring your arms alongside the hips with the palms turned upward.
4. Breathe and relax.

How to Come out of Viparita Karani, Prenatal Var.

1. Bend the knees, pushing the feet against the wall. Lift the hips, and shift and drop to the right.
2. Draw the right arm in to the chest.
3. Roll to the left.
4. Pause.
5. Prepare for what's next.

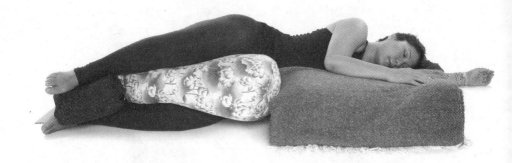

SIDE-LYING SAVASANA, PRENATAL VAR.
(SIDE-LYING CORPSE POSE, PRENATAL VAR.)

How to Move into Side-Lying Savasana, Prenatal Var.

1. Position two bolsters end to end on the mat, like a bed.
2. Place another blanket, if needed, on top of the bolster that the head and torso will rest on. This is needed if the elbow of the top arm needs to be more on the same plane as the shoulder.
3. Rest on the left side of the body with the bottom arm stretched overhead and a blanket folded as a meditation pad placed between that arm and the head.
4. Place the second bolster between the legs, and place a double-folded blanket folded in half and rolled between the ankles and feet to fill the space.
5. Rest the top arm on the top bolster.
6. Breathe and relax.

How to Come out of Side-Lying Savasana, Prenatal Var.

1. Allow movement to stir throughout the body.
2. Push against the floor with the right hand, and lift the body to an upright position.
3. Pause.
4. Prepare for what's next.

CONCLUSION

....

The light of wisdom that lives within us is so powerful it can turn winter into spring.

Our practice never ends. Life presents abundant opportunities to return to our yoga practice over and over. We all experience challenge and success, heartache and joy. Falling back on unhealthy habits keeps us trapped in our smaller selves and distances us from deeply taking charge of our self-care and well-being.

The Yapana BEING and STILL poses transform the way we see, experience, and accept things in ourselves, in others, and in the world around us. Yapana practice provides insight into the kind of mind and attitude needed for living a balanced life on and off the yoga mat:

Our practice offers us time to work hard and time to be soothed. The Yapana BEING and STILL segments cultivate a relaxed body and quiet mind and soothe our soul.

Our practice is now. Now. And now.

Namaste.

POSE INDEX

ABOUT THE AUTHOR

....

With gratitude, I stand on the shoulders of all my teachers. They have shared with me an abundance of knowledge and experience that has inspired me to explore and share the path of yoga with others.

Leeann Carey fell in love with yoga in the late 1970s and has never wavered in her passion to share the transformational benefits of this ancient yet timeless science of life. Leeann shares that knowledge today through Yapana restorative yoga therapy teacher-training programs and workshops and through Leeann Carey Yoga mentors across the United States and Canada.

In 1993, Leeann opened the first full-service yoga studio in her South Bay community in Southern California. There she developed important skills for operating a successful "yoga business" and went on to create a teacher-training school and the Yapana restorative yoga therapy program. Her eclectic blend of yoga appeals to a wide range of students and was forged over many years of study with gifted teachers, including Kofi Busia, Donna Farhi, Richard C. Miller, Erich Schiffmann, and Judith Lasater.

An ERYT-500 certified instructor, Leeann has mastered the traditional techniques and developed new approaches to serve and support all students — young or old, fit or physically challenged — to enrich their lives in body, mind, and spirit. She has applied her knowledge and experience to help professional athletes heal from injuries and improve their workouts and sports performance, including members of the World Champion Los Angeles Lakers and Olympic Gold Medal volleyball player Eric Fonoimoana.

For more information on Yapana practice, teacher training, and events, visit **YapanaYoga.com.**

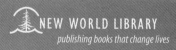